Exercise Biomechanics: Pathways to Improve Health

Exercise Biomechanics: Pathways to Improve Health

Guest Editors

Pedro Miguel Forte
José Eduardo Teixeira

MDPI

Basel • Beijing • Wuhan • Barcelona • Belgrade • Novi Sad • Cluj • Manchester

Guest Editors
Pedro Miguel Forte
Department of Sports
Higher Institute of
Educational Sciences of the
Douro
Penafiel
Portugal

José Eduardo Teixeira
Sports Science Department
Polytechnic of Cávado and
Ave
Guimarães
Portugal

Editorial Office
MDPI AG
Grosspeteranlage 5
4052 Basel, Switzerland

This is a reprint of the Special Issue, published open access by the journal *Healthcare* (ISSN 2227-9032), freely accessible at: https://www.mdpi.com/journal/healthcare/special_issues/K6SIT6RVY2.

For citation purposes, cite each article independently as indicated on the article page online and as indicated below:

Lastname, A.A.; Lastname, B.B. Article Title. *Journal Name* **Year**, *Volume Number*, Page Range.

ISBN 978-3-7258-7835-2 (Hbk)
ISBN 978-3-7258-7836-9 (PDF)
https://doi.org/10.3390/books978-3-7258-7836-9

Contents

Preface

This Reprint brings together a collection of scientific contributions that explores the role of exercise biomechanics in understanding and improving human health. The central aim is to provide an integrated perspective on how mechanical principles underpin movement, physical performance, and health-related outcomes across different populations and contexts.

Exercise biomechanics offers valuable tools to analyze human motion through the interaction of forces, joint mechanics, and neuromuscular function. The studies included in this Reprint reflect the growing relevance of combining experimental approaches with computational modeling to enhance the accuracy and applicability of biomechanical assessments. Such approaches contribute to a deeper understanding of movement efficiency, load distribution, and injury mechanisms.

The Reprint also highlights the practical implications of biomechanical knowledge in areas such as physical activity promotion, rehabilitation, and sports performance. By translating scientific findings into applied settings, biomechanics supports the development of evidence-based strategies aimed at optimizing performance while reducing the risk of injury.

This Reprint is addressed to researchers, clinicians, and professionals in the fields of health, sport, and human movement sciences. It aims to foster interdisciplinary collaboration and to encourage the continued integration of biomechanics into health-oriented research and practice, contributing to improved quality of life and long-term well-being.

Pedro Miguel Forte and José Eduardo Teixeira
Guest Editors

healthcare

MDPI

Editorial

Exercise Biomechanics for Health: Evaluating Lifelong Activities for Well-Being

Pedro Forte [1,2,3,*] and José E. Teixeira [2,3,4]

1 CI-ISCE, Higher Institute of Educational Sciences of the Douro, 4560-708 Penafiel, Portugal
2 Department of Sport Sciences, Polytechnic of Bragança, 5300-253 Bragança, Portugal
3 Research Centre in Sports Sciences, Health, and Human Development, 6201-001 Covilhã, Portugal
4 Department of Sport Sciences, Polytechnic of Guarda, 6300-559 Guarda, Portugal
* Correspondence: pedromiguel.forte@iscedouro.pt

Keywords: biomechanics; load; lifelong; performance; health

1. Exercise Biomechanics for Health

Biomechanics is a multidisciplinary study of the mechanical laws and principles that govern human movement and the functioning of biological systems [1]. In the context of physical activity, exercise and physical fitness, biomechanics plays a crucial role in understanding the most efficient and effective ways to improve health and well-being. In addition, biomechanics aim to improve athletes' performance as well as the movement efficiency of the whole population, leading to a better quality of life. To that end, concerns about optimal economy of movement, strength, power, stability, postural alignment, range of motion and athletic performance are some of the most important topics to address in the study of exercise biomechanics [2].

By studying optimal movement patterns, we aim to understand proper movement patterns and techniques, with the objective to reduce the risk of injury and improve exercise efficiency, thus leading to better health outcomes [3]. Optimal movement refers to the most efficient and effective ways to perform a specific exercise or movement in terms of reducing the risk of injury and illness, as well as improving exercise efficiency, thus leading to better health outcomes [4]. In this field of research, body alignment, joint angles, muscle activation patterns and the transfer of force through the body are variables to consider when assessing optimal movement. For this purpose, specialists (healthcare technicians and medical doctors, including physiotherapists, rehabilitation nurses and medical doctors in sports medicine and physiatry; as well as fitness technicians, including exercise physiologists, fitness instructors and strength and conditioning coaches) may use this information to design and apply evidence-based exercises in training and technician programs.

Exercise biomechanics constantly deal with strength levels, stability and postural alignment. Physical exercise can improve strength and stability, whereby specialists may help individuals to understand and correct posture and misalignments and control strength and stability levels, thus contributing to reducing the risk of injury and illness [5]. Postural imbalances are usually related to stress on the joints and muscles, leading to pain, discomfort and functional decline. Thus, proper alignment of the joints during exercise is crucial to reduce the risk of injury and improve overall function and health. In addition, improved flexibility and range of motion is another topic of relevance in this field; specialists can design different stretching exercises to improve flexibility that target specific areas of the body [6,7]. This may reduce pain and musculoskeletal disorders and, thus, improve overall health and quality of life. Concerning optimal athletic performance, technique efficiency is paramount during strength and power training exercises, as well as during sports-specific sports-based movements [8,9]. This helps to minimize the risk of injury and ensures the efficient use of energy and muscular contribution, leading to improved performance (lower cost for better performance). The biomechanical kinetic and kinematic parameters will help with design programs and allow them to increase power and explosiveness, and, thus, to enhance coordination, reaction time and overall performance.

Proper exercise biomechanics involves the correct form and technique in different joint and anatomical planes during physical activity, exercise and sports activities to ensure that the joints, muscles and bones are moving in a safe and efficient manner. In terms of health and wellness, where physical activity plays an important role, different types of physical activity may require different biomechanical techniques as well as physiological and physical demands. Thus, a healthcare professional or trained fitness professional should be consulted before starting a new exercise program for assessment, prescription and control. The biomechanics of the exercise provide a better understanding of distinct physical limitations, allowing individuals to adjust their exercise program accordingly. The literature continues to call for exercise biomechanics research related to health. Thus, a call for research that emphasizes the importance of methods and information to improve the practices of coaches and players remains important [10,11].

Contributions that, from a biomechanical viewpoint, will explain and examine several biomechanics-related topics in exercise and sports. Discussion of useful applications and/or many other topics of interest has been reported; physical activity, rehabilitation, fitness and competitive sport are appreciated by the exercise biomechanics research community. For that, testing methods, equipment and evaluation techniques will allow us to improve the knowledge required to monitor and evaluate the biomechanical load in health-related physical activity, exercise and sports practice.

2. Lifelong Biomechanics

Lifelong biomechanical kinetic and kinematic analyses are the focus of studies on human movement patterns and forces, as well as their repercussions on the body (physical and physiological impact) throughout time [9]. By analyzing these patterns and the mechanics of human movement, individuals can better understand how their physical activity and exercise habits affect their health and physical condition, as well as how they contribute to general well-being [12]. Biomechanical overload can lead to overuse injuries, joint degeneration and other chronic conditions. On the other hand, a lack of biomechanical load can lead to decreased strength, balance, flexibility and physical function. To assess the effects of biomechanical load on health, it is important to consider a variety of factors, especially physical and exercise methodology principles such as intensity, duration and frequency. Additionally, the individual's age, health status and physical abilities should be also considered in biomechanics [13,14]. By taking these factors into consideration, individuals can better understand the effects of their physical activity and exercise on their body over time and make informed decisions about their exercise program to optimize their physical fitness, health and well-being.

Tools and technologies will help researchers and practitioners to better understand the mechanics of human movement, and can be used to improve exercise programs, injury prevention strategies and overall athletic performance. Testing equipment, instruments, gears and software used in the field of exercise biomechanics will allow researchers to assess and analyze human movement. Some of the most commonly used techniques are motion capture systems, which analyze the movement of joints, bones and muscles and can be used with sensors, cameras or wearable devices [9]. Among the various instruments, force and pressure plates are used to measure the force and power generated during movement as well as the ground reaction forces and pressure distributions during the movement [15]. Electromyography (EMG) is used to measure muscle activation and electrical activity during movement [16]; goniometers and inclinometers are used to assess joint angles/range of motion [16]; the simulation software allows for evaluation of human movement in a virtual environment, considering kinetic and kinematic variables in assumed conditions (controlling inputs) [17]; and, finally, wearable devices, such as accelerometers and gyroscopes, are used to monitor and record movement data in real time [18]. Along these lines, additional research is required in order to test more recent and different methodologies to assess the lifelong biomechanical load, as technology, information and data are becoming increasingly fast, user-friendly and accessible.

3. A Call for Research Topics

Finally, exercise biomechanics is a critical area for study and research that provides valuable insights into how physical activity, exercise and sports affect the body and health. The principles of exercise biomechanics are rooted in the mechanics of human movement and the effects of physical activity and exercise on the body over time. The study of biomechanics allows us to optimize athletic performance and prevent injury-related disability. By understanding the mechanics of human movement, individuals can design effective exercise programs that target specific physical imbalances and impairments to improve their physical function and general well-being. Specifically, health-focused biomechanics is a specific and important research field to produce scientific evidence for overall health and well-being. Several methods are available for assessing biomechanical variables in different contexts related to health and well-being, each with its own advantages and limitations. The most effective method will depend on the specific information desired and the context in which the assessment is being conducted.

Exercise biomechanics is a complex and multidisciplinary field that provides valuable insights into how physical activity, exercise and sports affect body function and health. By understanding the principles of biomechanics, individuals can make informed decisions about their exercise program to optimize their physical health and well-being. Contributions in the form of research papers on sports biomechanics-related topics and their useful applications, as well as those discussing other topics of interest, such as physical activity, rehabilitation, physical fitness and competitive sport, will lead to improvement in the scientific knowledge and practices in this research field.

Author Contributions: Conceptualization, P.F. and J.E.T.; writing—original draft preparation, P.F. and J.E.T.; writing—review and editing, P.F. and J.E.T. All authors have read and agreed to the published version of the manuscript.

Conflicts of Interest: The authors declare no conflict of interest.

References

1. Knudson, D. *Fundamentals of Biomechanics*; Springer: Berlin/Heidelberg, Germany, 2021. [CrossRef]
2. Forte, P.; Neiva, H.P.; Marinho, D.A. Sports Biomechanics: Monitoring Health and Performance. *J. Men's Health* **2021**, *17*, 4–6. [CrossRef]
3. Glazier, P.S.; Mehdizadeh, S. Challenging Conventional Paradigms in Applied Sports Biomechanics Research. *Sport. Med.* **2019**, *49*, 171–176. [CrossRef] [PubMed]
4. Wallace, B.; Kernozek, T. Self-Efficacy Theory Applied to Undergraduate Biomechanics Instruction. *J. Hosp. Leis. Sport Tour. Educ.* **2017**, *20*, 10–15. [CrossRef]
5. Alves, M.E.; Marinho, D.A.; Carneiro, D.N.; Alves, J.; Forte, P.; Nevill, A.M.; Morais, J.E. A Visual Scan Analysis Protocol for Postural Assessment at School in Young Students. *Int. J. Environ. Res. Public Health* **2020**, *17*, 2915. [CrossRef] [PubMed]
6. Nagai, T.; Abt, J.P.; Sell, T.C.; Clark, N.C.; Smalley, B.W.; Wirt, M.D.; Lephart, S.M. Neck Proprioception, Strength, Flexibility, and Posture in Pilots with and Without Neck Pain History. *Aviat. Space Environ. Med.* **2014**, *85*, 529–535. [CrossRef] [PubMed]
7. Moezy, A.; Sepehrifar, S.; Dodaran, M.S. The Effects of Scapular Stabilization Based Exercise Therapy on Pain, Posture, Flexibility and Shoulder Mobility in Patients with Shoulder Impingement Syndrome: A Controlled Randomized Clinical Trial. *Med. J. Islam. Repub. Iran* **2014**, *28*, 87. [PubMed]
8. Morriën, F.; Taylor, M.J.D.; Hettinga, F.J. Biomechanics in Paralympics: Implications for Performance. *Int. J. Sport. Physiol. Perform.* **2017**, *12*, 578–589. [CrossRef] [PubMed]
9. Hood, S.; McBain, T.; Portas, M.; Spears, L. Measurement in Sports Biomechanics. *Meas. Control* **2012**, *45*, 182–186. [CrossRef]
10. Van Emmerik, R.E.A.; Ducharme, S.W.; Amado, A.C.; Hamill, J. Comparing Dynamical Systems Concepts and Techniques for Biomechanical Analysis. *J. Sport Health Sci.* **2016**, *5*, 3–13. [CrossRef] [PubMed]
11. Choppin, S.; Wheat, J. The Potential of the Microsoft Kinect in Sports Analysis and Biomechanics. *Sport. Technol.* **2013**, *6*, 78–85. [CrossRef]
12. Pascoe, M.; Bailey, A.P.; Craike, M.; Carter, T.; Patten, R.; Stepto, N.; Parker, A. Physical Activity and Exercise in Youth Mental Health Promotion: A Scoping Review. *BMJ Open Sport Exerc. Med.* **2020**, *6*, e000677. [CrossRef] [PubMed]

13. Doeven, S.H.; Brink, M.S.; Huijgen, B.C.H.; de Jong, J.; Lemmink, K.A.P.M. High Match Load's Relation to Decreased Well-Being During an Elite Women's Rugby Sevens Tournament. *Int. J. Sport. Physiol. Perform.* **2019**, *14*, 1036–1042. [CrossRef] [PubMed]
14. Apte, S.; Prigent, G.; Stöggl, T.; Martínez, A.; Snyder, C.; Gremeaux-Bader, V.; Aminian, K. Biomechanical Response of the Lower Extremity to Running-Induced Acute Fatigue: A Systematic Review. *Front. Physiol.* **2021**, *12*, 646042. [CrossRef] [PubMed]
15. Barbosa, J.; Marques, M.C.; Forte, P.; Santos, C.C.; Neiva, H.P.; Izquierdo, M.; Marinho, D.A. Effects of a Modified Backpack Model on Ground Reaction Forces in Children of Different Ages during Walking and Running. *J. Men's Health* **2022**, *18*, 109. [CrossRef]
16. Monteiro-Oliveira, B.B.; Coelho-Oliveira, A.C.; Paineiras-Domingos, L.L.; Sonza, A.; Sá-Caputo, D.d.C.d.; Bernardo-Filho, M. Use of Surface Electromyography to Evaluate Effects of Whole-Body Vibration Exercises on Neuromuscular Activation and Muscle Strength in the Elderly: A Systematic Review. *Disabil. Rehabil.* **2021**, *44*, 7368–7377. [CrossRef] [PubMed]
17. Forte, P.; Marinho, D.A.; Morais, J.E.; Morouço, P.G.; Barbosa, T.M. Estimation of Mechanical Power and Energy Cost in Elite Wheelchair Racing by Analytical Procedures and Numerical Simulations. *Comput. Methods Biomech. Biomed. Eng.* **2018**, *21*, 585–592. [CrossRef]
18. Teixeira, J.E.; Alves, A.R.; Ferraz, R.; Forte, P.; Leal, M.; Ribeiro, J.; Silva, A.J.; Barbosa, T.M.; Monteiro, A.M. Effects of Chronological Age, Relative Age, and Maturation Status on Accumulated Training Load and Perceived Exertion in Young Sub-Elite Football Players. *Front. Physiol.* **2022**, *13*, 547. [CrossRef] [PubMed]

healthcare

MDPI

Article

Biomechanical Effects of the MIND&GAIT Exercise Program on Sit-to-Stand and Marching in Place Motor Coordination in Institutionalized Older Adults: Implications for Functional Stability

Cristiana Mercê [1,2,3,4,*], Susana Alfaiate [1], Fátima Ramalho [1,2], David Catela [1,2,5] and Marco Branco [1,2,3,4]

1 Sport Sciences School of Rio Maior (ESDRM), Santarém Polytechnic University, Av. Dr. Mário Soares, 110, 2040-413 Rio Maior, Portugal; 090517001@esdrm.ipsantarem.pt (S.A.); fatimaramalho@esdrm.ipsantarem.pt (F.R.); catela@esdrm.ipsantarem.pt (D.C.); marcobranco@esdrm.ipsantarem.pt (M.B.)
2 Sport Physical Activity and Health Research & Innovation Center (SPRINT), Santarém Polytechnic University, Av. Dr. Mário Soares, 110, 2040-413 Rio Maior, Portugal
3 Physical Activity and Health—Life Quality Research Centre (CIEQV), Santarém Polytechnic University, Complexo Andaluz, Apart 279, 2001-904 Santarém, Portugal
4 Interdisciplinary Center for the Study of Human Performance (CIPER), Faculty of Human Kinetics, University of Lisbon, Cruz Quebrada-Dafundo, 1499-002 Lisboa, Portugal
5 Quality Education—Life Quality Research Centre (CIEQV), Santarém Polytechnic University, Complexo Andaluz, Apart 279, 2001-904 Santarém, Portugal
* Correspondence: cristianamerce@esdrm.ipsantarem.pt

Highlights

What are the main findings?

- The MIND&GAIT program generated positive trends in motor variability and unpredictability in sit-to-stand and marching-in-place tasks, despite no statistically significant changes.
- Results suggest improvements in adaptive motor coordination, particularly during the marching-in-place task, with shifts toward more flexible and divergent movement patterns.

What are the implications of the main findings?

- These biomechanical trends suggest that MIND&GAIT may enhance functional stability and adaptability to perturbations, mechanisms essential to fall prevention.
- These exploratory results support the inclusion of structured exercise programs like MIND&GAIT as a valuable strategy for reducing fall vulnerability in institutionalized older adults.

Abstract

Background: Motor decline associated with ageing compromises mobility, postural control and the ability, thereby increasing risk among older adults. Biomechanical characterization of movement, particularly using non-linear methods, offers a process-oriented approach capable of detecting subtle changes in motor coordination. The MIND&GAIT programme has previously demonstrated benefits in physical function in frail older individuals; however, its potential to improve motor coordination parameters that underpin fall risk remains insufficiently explored. **Objectives**: To analyse the impact of the MIND&GAIT program on motor coordination during sit-to-stand (STS) and walking tasks, two daily activities strongly associated with fall risk, using advanced non-linear and biomechanical metrics in institutionalized older adults. **Methods**: Fourteen institutionalized older adults (82.21 ± 7.14 years) participated. Three-dimensional acceleration and angular velocity were recorded using inertial sensors. Motor variability and predictability were quantified using the multivariate Lyapunov exponent (LyEM) and multivariate incremental entropy (MIE). STS (30 s) and walking-in-place (2 min) tasks were assessed pre- and post-intervention following a three-month, thrice-weekly programme. **Results**: Although no statistically significant differences emerged ($ps > 0.05$), trends were observed suggesting increases in LyEM during STS and in both MIE and LyEM during walking were found post-intervention. These exploratory findings may indicate enhanced motor complexity, stability and adaptability, features associated with reduced fall vulnerability. **Conclusions**: Despite the absence of statistical significance, the biomechanical trends observed suggest improvements in motor coordination patterns relevant to fall risk reduction in institutionalized older adults following the MIND&GAIT programme. These findings highlight the potential of structured exercise-based interventions for promoting safer movement behaviors in frail populations.

Keywords: older adults; inertial sensors; non-linear dynamics; motor variability; functional mobility; motor development; exercise; group fitness; health; fall risk

1. Introduction

Ageing affects the sensory systems involved in postural control, increasing whole-body instability and, in older adults, the likelihood of falls [1]. As sensory deficits accumulate with age, gait patterns also change, including greater variability and slower gait speed, which are associated with reduced ankle range of motion [2,3]. Gait is a gross motor task that requires balance, strength and coordination. For this reason, analyzing its spatio-temporal parameters, along with their variability, is essential for identifying pathologies and motor disorders [4,5]. The sit-to-stand movement is likewise a fundamental daily task, especially for older adults. It is crucial for maintaining independence, and numerous studies have demonstrated its association with lower-limb strength in older populations [1]. Similar to gait, difficulties in performing this movement can predict fall risk. These difficulties may arise from muscle weakness, balance impairments, joint limitations, or other physical constraints [6]. Physical inactivity is associated with poor motor control and reduced movement speed, whereas the practice of physical exercise can improve both functional fitness parameters and gait performance [7,8]. It therefore becomes pertinent to stimulate and assess not only the physical capacities of older adults, but also their coordinative abilities during everyday functional tasks.

In the fields of biomechanics and motor behavior research, several methodologies and instruments have been used [9]. Inertial Measurement Units (IMUs), stand out as key tools for movement analysis, providing three-dimensional data on angular velocity and linear acceleration. These small instruments, typically composed by triaxial magnetometers, accelerometers and gyroscopes, allow reliable quantification of functional tasks, such as balance assessments or impact transmission across body segments. IMUs are practical, easy to use, and support detailed examination of linear and angular movements, enabling the estimation of temporal, kinematic and dynamic parameters [9].

To achieve a deeper understanding of variability and stability patterns in movement, non-linear analytical measures have gained increasing relevance [10]. Entropy is a metric capable of quantifying and predicting irregularities in time series data, offering deeper and more complex insight into movement mechanisms. Non-linear analysis, particularly entropy, has proven to be an important tool for understanding the complexity of human

 https://doi.org/10.3390/healthcare14060770

movement. Unlike traditional linear analyses, which may fail to capture the richness of dynamic data, entropy provides a means to quantify irregularity and predictability in time series [11].

Multivariate Incremental Entropy (MIE) is highly effective for analyzing short signals or limited datasets, as it is particularly sensitive to subtle changes in the underlying structure, indicating higher or lower randomness and predictability in motor behavior [12]. Higher MIE values reflect greater unpredictability within the system, meaning lower predictability, which corresponds to an increased adaptive capacity when facing perturbations. Ageing is typically associated with a reduction in such adaptive capacities when responding to stability challenges [13,14]. Given that frail, institutionalized older adults commonly exhibit diminished postural control, slower compensatory reactions and higher susceptibility to balance disturbances, MIE becomes particularly relevant for capturing these subtle deficits [13]. By quantifying the degree of unpredictability in motor responses, MIE can differentiate between preserved and impaired adaptive capacity—information that traditional linear metrics often fail to detect in this population. Thus, MIE provides a sensitive framework to examine how ageing and frailty impact motor behavior dynamics and system stability, supporting the design of more targeted interventions to enhance adaptation in older populations.

The calculation of the Lyapunov exponent (LyE), also a non-linear metric, is widely recognized in dynamic systems analysis and is considered an efficient method for studying motor behavior because it allows the assessment of the variability and adaptability of a system when exposed to perturbations [15,16]. This technique has been used in several tests, including sit-to-stand, finger tapping, and gait tasks [11]. The computation of the maximum Lyapunov exponent enables the analysis of complex systems by examining whether system trajectories converge (i.e., negative values) or diverge (i.e., positive values), thereby assessing variability and behavioral stability. Higher LyE values reflect greater variability in behavior, as well as greater adaptive capacity when the system is exposed to perturbations [17]. Nevertheless, it is important, to distinguish adaptive variability, characterized by flexible and functional adjustments to perturbations, from pathological instability, which reflects excessive, uncontrolled divergence of system trajectories. While moderate increases in LyE suggest healthy adaptability, disproportionately high values may indicate compromised motor control and instability rather than functional responsiveness [18].

Bearing in mind that non-linear measures such as MIE and the LyE are sensitively capture the complexity, variability, and adaptive capacity of motor control [14,17]. And that within the ageing process the changes in fundamental tasks as gait and sit-to-stand can reflect functional instability and greater vulnerability to perturbations and falls [1]. It is pertinent to evaluate interventions that act directly on these coordination determinants. MIND&GAIT is a multicomponent program validated for older adults [19], designed to improve functional fitness and mobility in seniors by combining structured physical exercise (i.e., lower-limb strength, balance, coordination, and mobility) with progressive cognitive stimulation. Through tasks and progressions that demand efficient spatiotemporal organization of movement, postural adjustment, and adaptive responses to perturbations, the program inherently targets mechanisms associated with fall prevention. Nevertheless, despite the established relevance of non-linear metrics for understanding motor coordination, there is a clear research gap: no studies to date have examined whether MIND&GAIT produces measurable changes in non-linear motor coordination metrics, as MIE or LyE, in institutionalized older adults. This limits current understanding of how multicomponent training may influence system adaptability and stability at a dynamical level.

 https://doi.org/10.3390/healthcare14060770

To address this gap, and following the need to characterize changes in motor coordination in ecologically valid tasks using inertial sensors (IMUs) and non-linear metrics, the present study aimed to analyze the effects of the MIND&GAIT exercise program on gross motor coordination, through variability (LyE) and predictability (Entropy), in the sit-to-stand (STS) and marching in place tasks.

2. Materials and Methods

2.1. Study Design

A quasi-experimental design with a single experimental group and a quantitative approach. The physical exercise program included 37 sessions in total, during 12 weeks with three sessions per week. The physical sessions were performed at light to moderate intensity. The protocol included three phases: (i) pre-intervention assessment, (ii) intervention, and (iii) post-intervention assessment.

This study was designed to prioritize a process-oriented analysis of motor coordination using nonlinear metrics (LyEM and MIE) during ecologically valid tasks (STS and marching-in-place). Assessments were conducted within one week before and after the 12-week intervention (37 sessions). Sample size was constrained by the single-center exploratory scope; no a priori power calculation was performed. Once all residents who met the eligibility criteria agreed to participate, it was not possible to form an equivalent control group. Deliberately excluding eligible participants would not have been ethically acceptable in this context. In this sense, a single-group quasi-experimental design was adopted. Without a control group, threats to internal validity (e.g., learning effects, day-to-day variability, health fluctuations, regression to the mean) cannot be excluded; we standardized assessor, setting, and sensor placement to mitigate procedural variance.

Ethical approval for this study was obtained from the Ethics Committee of the Polytechnic University of Santarém (approval number 10-2024 ESDRM).

Reporting followed the TREND statement for non-randomized evaluations and relevant STROBE items for observational reporting; a completed checklist is available upon request.

2.2. Sample

The program was implemented at an elderly day center located in a city in central Portugal. All residents who met the inclusion criteria were invited to participate, totaling an initial number of 21 older adults. Due to hospitalization (n = 1), change of institution (n = 4), death (n = 1), and worsening of pre-existing pathologies (n = 1), only 14 participants completed the program and its assessments. Therefore, this was a convenience sample.

The final sample was composed by 14 older adults of both sexes (10 women), aged between 70 and 93 years (M = 82.69 $\pm$ 6.81 years). Inclusion criteria included non-participation in other physical exercise programs, the absence of neurodegenerative diseases, and no contraindications for physical exercise [7].

2.3. MIND&GAIT Program

The MIND&GAIT programme, previously developed and validated for frail older adults [19], was adapted in the present study to the institutionalized elderly population. To optimize its applicability and ensure sufficient training stimulus in this context, the weekly frequency was increased from the original two to three sessions per week. The program included 37 sessions over 12 weeks with three sessions a week, each lasting 45 to 60 min.

The programme focused on functional capacity such as postural stability, lower-limb strength, balance, agility and aerobic endurance. All exercises were structured progressively and adjusted to each participant's individual abilities. Sessions' intensity was monitored

https://doi.org/10.3390/healthcare14060770

using the Modified Borg Rating of Perceived Exertion, and targeting that the training remained within light (1–4) to moderate (5–6) effort levels.

The program included aerobic, balance, strength and flexibility exercises. It also included a more playful aspect to promote socializing and the well-being of the participants, while also emphasizing posture stability, strength, balance, agility and aerobic capacity. All exercises and games were performed with an intensity adjusted to each participant's abilities.

In terms of its periodization, the program included an initial adaptation and learning phase, which sought to increase body awareness (i.e., acquisition of neutral alignment, pelvic and scapular alignment, control of spinal mobility), identify breathing patterns, and train posture and balance, training weight distribution across both feet. As the program progressed and in line with the participants' progress, the intensity was gradually increased. The sessions lasted approximately 45 to 60 min and were divided into three parts: (i) warm-up, 5 to 10 min, including body awareness, breathing, joint warm-up; (ii) main phase: 25–35 min, aerobic, strength, and functional training including balance; (iii) cool down and stretching, 5–10 min [19]. The end of the sessions always included a game, a dance, coordination exercises or object manipulation. Table 1 below shows the structure of the classes.

Table 1. Systematization of the class structure.

Phases	Scope	Aims	Content	Method
Warm up 5 to 10 min	Gradual transition from the pre-exercise phase (rest) to the exercise phase	Gradual warming up of muscles and joints Preparation for exercise	Body awareness Weight control through support Breathing General joint mobility	Light intensity Lower and upper limbs Local joint mobility General joint mobility Static stretching
Main Phase 30 to 35 min	Aerobic training	Improvement of cardiorespiratory capacity Coordination	Walking Coordination and sensorimotor exercises (visual and auditory stimuli) Rhythm Agility Laterality	Dynamic exercises HR [1]—range of 40 to 50% of maximum heart rate Borg scale 3 to 6 (scale of 0 to 10)
	Strength training	Ability to produce tension in a specific muscle group Large muscle groups Work Muscle strength ADLs [2] Replication	Lower muscles/upper muscles Agonist/antagonist Flexor muscles/extensor muscles Core activation	5 to 8 exercises 8 to 12 repetitions 2 to 3 sets 50 to 60% of 1 RM [3] 2 min recovery
Cool down/Stretching 5 to 10 min	Transition between exercise and rest Flexibility Balance	Decreased heart and respiratory rates Muscle relaxation	Stretching, relaxation, and breathing Joint mobility	Calm music Interactive game Slow movements Static/dynamic stretching Comfortable joint movement, without causing pain

[1] Heart rate, [2] activities of daily life, [3] one-repetition maximum.

https://doi.org/10.3390/healthcare14060770

All sessions were delivered by a certified exercise professional with specific training in the MIND&GAIT programme and prior experience delivering exercise sessions to frail and institutionalized older adults. At the time of implementation, the instructor was a Master's student specializing in this field and had received dedicated training from the programme's development team, ensuring fidelity to the original protocol and safe, correct execution of all exercises. All session plans and Borg RPE ranges were systematically logged to monitor fidelity.

2.4. Motor Coordination Assessment

To assess gross motor coordination in daily life representative tasks, the 2 min marching test and the sit-to-stand (STS) test were selected, both part of the functional battery proposed by Rikli & Jones [20] and validated for evaluating physical fitness in older adults. The 2 min marching test consisted of marching in place for 2 min, raising the knee to the midpoint between the patella and the iliac crest; this point was individually identified for each participant and visibly marked at the testing site to ensure uniform execution. The marching-in-place test was selected because it is a validated protocol for older adults within the Rikli and Jones [20] functional battery and offers greater safety and feasibility in frail, institutionalized populations. This dynamic task captures rhythmic and variability-related components of gait while ensuring a controlled environment and minimizing fall risk. Performing the task in place also enhances signal standardization required for non-linear analysis. Nevertheless, it is acknowledged that its ecological validity is lower than that of overground walking. The STS test consisted of standing up and sitting down on a chair as many times as possible within 30 s, with the arms crossed over the chest [20].

Three-dimensional linear acceleration and angular velocity data were collected using a small inertial sensor equipped with a gyroscope (MPU 9250, Invensense, TDK Corporation, San Jose, CA, USA) [11]. All tests were administered by the same evaluators and in the same location to ensure procedural consistency. For both tasks, the sensor was positioned 10 cm above the anatomical landmark tibiale laterale. This placement was chosen to minimize soft-tissue artefacts resulting from displacement of the skin and surrounding tissues during knee flexion and extension, while maintaining a stable bony reference [9,11].

Data acquisition was performed using a custom software application developed by the authors in Python 3.12.10 with an HTML-based graphical interface and executed on a Windows 11 operating system. The application was designed to receive and store inertial sensor data transmitted wirelessly via Wi-Fi from the IMU devices. Data were transmitted using the UDP protocol through a dedicated communication port and recorded in real time without any preprocessing or modification of the original signal. The application stored the timestamps generated by the sensors together with the transmitted inertial measurements, preserving the original temporal structure of the signal. The acquired data were saved as plain text files (.txt) and subsequently used for offline processing and analysis. Subsequent signal processing and nonlinear analyses were conducted in MATLAB R2025a [11,21].

The data collected by the sensors were transmitted via Wi-Fi to a laptop computer using dedicated software, then exported to an Excel file and processed using a custom routine developed in MATLAB [11,21]. In this routine, the signal sampling frequency was determined from the time vector as the inverse of the mean sampling interval and was: (i) visually inspected and plotted for manual trimming before and after task execution; (ii) the trimmed raw signal was preprocessed using an adaptive band-pass filtering procedure. For each axis independently, a Fast Fourier Transform (FFT) was computed to obtain the single-sided amplitude spectrum. Frequencies below 0.1 Hz and above the Nyquist frequency were excluded. Dominant frequency components were identified using a peak detection algorithm with a threshold set at 1% of the maximum spectral amplitude. Lower

https://doi.org/10.3390/healthcare14060770

and upper cutoff frequencies were adaptively defined by expanding the minimum and maximum detected peak frequencies by ±1 Hz. The resulting passband was constrained within 0.1–5 Hz to ensure physiologically plausible movement frequencies. The signal was then filtered using a 4th-order Butterworth band-pass filter, with cutoff frequencies normalized to the Nyquist frequency, followed by a zero-phase forward–backward filtering to prevent phase distortion and preserve the temporal structure of the signal [22,23]; (iii) For each axis, local maxima and minima were identified using a finding peaks function, applying a minimum inter-peak distance of 0.5 s and a prominence threshold set at 20% of the signal range to reduce spurious detections, with visual confirmation of the time series for verification; (iv) the filtered triaxial inertial signal was transformed to absolute values, and no other normalizations were made to the signal; (v) Phase-space parameters were estimated as follows: the time delay (τ) was defined as the first lag where the autocorrelation dropped below 0.1 (up to a maximum lag of 500 samples), the embedding dimension (m) was obtained using an optimized false-nearest-neighbors approach with maximum dimension set to 4, and the tolerance parameter (R) was estimated via an optimized fraction-based procedure. The reconstruction of system dynamics from delay coordinates is based on embedding theory [24], with FNN used for practical embedding dimension estimation [25]. Final multivariate parameters were combined using the maximum τ and m across axes and the minimum R across axes. (vi) Multivariate Incremental Entropy was computed over sliding windows whose length and step were defined from the mean cycle period estimated from the detected peaks, ensuring windowing consistent with task periodicity; (vii) for each recorded trial, the multivariate largest Lyapunov exponent (LyEM) was estimated from the triaxial inertial signal (X, Y, Z) simultaneously, using a Wolf-based approach to quantify divergence of nearby trajectories in phase space and capture the dynamics' sensitivity to initial conditions [26].

Approximately 30 min before testing, the sensors were calibrated using the IMU-DataReceiver software Version 1.0, which performs the initial signal processing.

During data collection, participants initiated the movement a few seconds after sensor activation. The analyzed movement segments were extracted from the first acceleration peak, corresponding to the start of the task (first extension to stand up in the STS test or first step in the marching task), to the last acceleration peak recorded for each task.

Similarly, Multivariate Incremental Entropy (MIE) was calculated according to established procedures in the literature [12] and adjusted across all axes, thus representing the multivariate complexity and predictability of the signal.

2.5. Data Treatment

Statistical analysis was performed using the Statistical Package for the Social Sciences software (version 29, SPSS Science, Chicago, IL, USA). Descriptive statistics were calculated to characterize the sample and all variables under study. The Shapiro–Wilk normality test was applied. According to the normality of the variables, paired *t*-tests or Wilcoxon tests were used to examine significant changes in multivariate incremental entropy and multivariate Lyapunov measures in the marching in place and STS tasks between pre- and post-intervention assessments. Effect sizes were calculated to complement the non-parametric analyses. For the Wilcoxon signed-rank tests, effect size (r) was derived using the formula $r = Z/\sqrt{N}$, in line with recommended procedures for non-parametric paired comparisons [27]. Magnitude was interpreted according to Cohen's benchmarks (small = 0.10, medium = 0.30, large = 0.50).

https://doi.org/10.3390/healthcare14060770

3. Results

The implementation of the program comprised 37 exercise sessions, and the participants' adherence and retention were exceptionally high. The participants attended on average 35.96 ± 1.56 sessions. Among the fourteen older adults, eight attended all sessions, four attended 35 sessions, one attended 34 sessions, and one attended 32 sessions.

Variability (LyEM) and unpredictability (MIE), two variables that allow the assessment of motor behavior, were evaluated in both the sit-to-stand (STS) and marching-in-place (MIP) tests both pre- and post-intervention. No significant differences were observed (all $ps > 0.05$). Nevertheless, increases in mean values were noted for LyEM in the STS test, as well as for both MIE and LyEM in the gait test, as presented in Table 2.

Table 2. Presentation of the descriptive and inferential statistics for multivariate incremental entropy (MIE) and multivariate Lyapunov (LyEM) measures across the two tasks, sit-to-stand (STS) and gait, and for the pre- and post-intervention assessments.

Tasks	Variable_Assessment	M	SD	Med	Min	Max	Tendency	*p*	*r*
STS	MIE_Pre- MIE_Post-	0.015 0.010	0.022 0.008	0.006 0.010	0.000 0.000	0.081 0.029	↓	0.753	0.084
	LyEM_Pre- LyEM_Post-	0.195 0.624	0.326 1.804	0.052 0.025	−0.003 −0.009	1.123 6.785	↑	0.594	0.142
MIP	MIE_Pre- MIE_Post-	0.052 0.088	0.058 0.092	0.021 0.087	0.000 0.000	0.158 0.284	↑	0.347	0.251
	LyEM_Pre- LyEM_Post-	0.039 0.307	0.083 0.678	0.016 0.035	−0.086 0.012	0.237 2.362	↑	0.182	0.357

M—mean, SD—standard deviation, Med—median, Min—minimum, Max—maximum, Pre—pre-intervention, Post—post-intervention, ↓—decrease from pre- to post-intervention, ↑—increase from pre- to post-intervention.

To complement the non-significant inferential results, effect sizes (r) from the Wilcoxon tests were calculated. These results indicated small effects in the STS task (MIE: $r = 0.084$; LyEM: $r = 0.142$) and small-to-moderate effects in the marching-in-place task (MIE: $r = 0.251$; LyEM: $r = 0.357$), suggesting slight but non-negligible magnitudes of change.

4. Discussion

The present study aimed to evaluate the effect of the MIND&GAIT program on motor coordination during the sit-to-stand (STS) and 2 min walking (marching in place) tests. Different methodologies may be used to assess motor coordination, including more traditional approaches such as phase plot analysis [28,29], as well as more innovative approaches such as nonlinear methods. Among nonlinear methods, the study of variability through multivariate Lyapunov Exponents (LyEM) and predictability through Multivariate Incremental Entropy (MIE) are two of the most widely recommended tools [12,15,17,30]. Importantly, these nonlinear variables are particularly relevant in a fall-prevention framework once they provide information about movement adaptability and the capacity to respond to perturbations, two key determinants of functional stability in older adults [10,31]. Although the present study focused exclusively on process-oriented nonlinear metrics, these measures are conceptually linked to more product-oriented and traditional indicators of functional mobility. Greater movement variability and complexity, when organized adaptively, have been associated with better performance in tasks such as gait speed, transitional movements, and balance recovery [31,32]. In this sense, increases in LyEM or MIE may reflect underlying mechanisms that support functional outcomes like safer gait or more efficient sit-to-stand performance. While we did not analyze clinical performance indicators in this manuscript, these relationships will be explored in detail in a separate study using the

 https://doi.org/10.3390/healthcare14060770

linear outputs collected with the same protocol. In addition to improving older adults' general health, physical exercise (PE) offers benefits for physical fitness, namely endurance, mobility, agility, speed, and motor coordination, a key factor for preventing the loss of functional capacities and dependency [33,34]. A lack of coordinative abilities leads to instability, which increases with aging and contributes to one of the major factors underlying loss of independence in older adults: falls. These events often result in physical and psychological impairments [35]. Gait stability depends on the individual's ability to maintain balance in the presence of disturbances. In the MIP task, both nonlinear indicators increased from pre- to post-intervention, with small-to-moderate effect sizes. Exactly, MIE increased from 0.052 to 0.088 and LyEM from 0.039 to 0.307, suggesting a tendency toward greater movement complexity and dynamic variability in the lower-limb movement pattern. From a biomechanical perspective, rhythmic stepping requires continuous regulation of limb oscillation, foot placement, and the transition between support and swing phases to maintain dynamic balance. Because the inertial sensor was positioned above the tibiale laterale, the recorded signal primarily reflects the dynamics of the distal lower-limb segment during stepping. In this context, the observed increases in MIE and LyEM may indicate a greater capacity to adapt the temporal organization and variability of lower-limb motion, which may be compatible with more flexible coordinative control during locomotor-like activity. These effects were more evident in MIP than in STS, which is consistent with the greater rhythmic and balance-related demands of the stepping task.

Dynamic balance and lower-limb coordination are particularly important when responding to unexpected situations [36]. Structured and supervised PE can also enhance lower-limb muscle strength, playing an essential role in the maintenance and improvement of functional capacity [37]. Given that falls often occur during transitional movements (e.g., rising from a chair) and during walking when unexpected perturbations arise, examining STS and marching in place (MIP) through variability and predictability metrics may help to capture subtle changes in functional stability that are not always detected by conventional outcomes. From a biomechanical perspective, the STS task involves a coordinated transition from a stable seated posture to upright standing, requiring forward displacement of the center of mass followed by extension of the lower-limb joints. This movement requires precise temporal coordination between load transfer, ankle and knee extension, and stabilization during seat-off. Because of the location of the inertial sensor, the recorded signal primarily reflects the dynamics of the distal lower-limb segment during this transition. In this context, the nonlinear metrics may capture subtle changes in the temporal organization and variability of the lower-limb movement pattern during the load-transfer and extension phases of STS. The observed increase in LyEM together with the small variation observed in MIE may therefore be compatible with slight modifications in the coordinative control of the lower limb during the postural transition, potentially reflecting a movement pattern that preserves adaptability while maintaining an organized temporal structure of the task.

From this perspective, it would be expected that older adults participating in the MIND&GAIT program would show increases in variability and unpredictability. However, contrary to the hypotheses, no statistically significant differences were found in any variable or task under analysis. Despite the lack of statistical significance, the effect sizes provide additional insight into the magnitude of the observed changes. In the STS task, effect sizes were small (r = 0.084–0.142), whereas MIP presented small-to-moderate magnitudes (r = 0.251–0.357). These values reinforce the presence of subtle but directionally consistent improvements, particularly in MIP, which align with the expected sensitivity of non-linear metrics to capture early adaptations in motor coordination. Importantly, these effect-size patterns also indicate that the STS task did not exhibit comparable direc-

 https://doi.org/10.3390/healthcare14060770

tional trends, especially regarding entropy, where mean MIE values decreased rather than increased. From a conceptual standpoint, the relationship between variability/entropy and functional performance is non-linear; consequently, increases in LyEM or MIE do not inherently denote "better" control. Depending on task demands, the amplitude and organization of fluctuations, greater variability can indicate either adaptive flexibility or excess noise/instability [38,39]. We therefore interpret the present changes as compatible with early adaptations in coordinative behavior predominantly in the MIP task, where increases were observed in both LyEM and MIE. In contrast, the STS task did not show a clear or consistent directional pattern, particularly for MIE, whose mean values decreased from pre- to post-intervention. Nevertheless, despite the lack of statistical significance, patterns of improvement in motor coordination can be observed. These improvements appear primarily in the MIP task, which showed increases in mean and maximum variability and unpredictability. For the STS task, only LyEM exhibited an increase in mean values, whereas MIE demonstrated a slight reduction, indicating that adaptations in this task were weaker or not directionally consistent. The Lyapunov Exponent quantifies a system's ability to mitigate small perturbations, with higher values indicating faster divergence of nearby trajectories in the reconstructed state space, which may reflect increased sensitivity of the movement dynamics to small perturbations and potentially greater adaptability to changing task demands [10,17]. Within an exploratory fall-prevention framework, these increases are better interpreted as changes consistent with improved regulation when challenged with small destabilizing events, rather than as evidence of functional benefits (e.g., fall prevention) per se. At the same time, it should be acknowledged that "more variability" is not universally beneficial; in frail older adults, excessively high or poorly organized variability can reflect impaired control [39]. Therefore, the observed post-intervention increases are best interpreted as potentially reflecting greater adaptability, rather than instability, especially in the MIP task, which is accompanied by concurrent trends in entropy and changes in LyE sign (negative to positive) suggestive of more flexible dynamics [10,16,17].

Among older adults, this adaptive capacity tends to decline with aging, reducing interactions among system components, as well as overall variability and complexity [40]. Thus, the observed increase in mean LyE may be interpreted as an indicator of improved motor coordination. Another supporting indicator is the reduction in negative LyE values. In the pre-intervention assessment, negative LyE values were found in both tests, reflecting a convergent and less adaptable system [10,17]. After the intervention, a slight reduction in LyE negativity was found in the STS test, and a notable improvement in the MIP test, which exhibited a positive LyE, characteristic of more divergent and adaptable systems. From a clinical standpoint, a shift toward more adaptable (divergent) dynamics during MIP may be meaningful because the ability to face perturbations without settling into rigid patterns is closely linked to safer locomotion and reduced balance loss. In contrast, the STS task showed only minimal LyE changes, with no accompanying increase in entropy, suggesting weaker or less consistent adaptive reorganization.

Similarly, higher MIE values indicate greater complexity and uncertainty in the system being analyzed. This implies lower predictability and higher variability, suggesting a more dynamic and adaptable system [12,40]. During senescence, motor behavior, including MIP, becomes more regular and less adaptable [12]. Just as muscle tissues become more "rigid" with aging, coordinative abilities also deteriorate, typically resulting in lower MIE values. The high variability observed in certain nonlinear parameters likely reflects inter-individual heterogeneity within this frail institutionalized sample. Such variability is expected in cohorts with diverse functional profiles and may also indicate the influence of individual outliers. These factors should be considered when interpreting dispersion patterns in LyEM and MIE. Accordingly, the observed post-intervention trends toward

https://doi.org/10.3390/healthcare14060770

higher MIE values may be viewed as compatible with enhanced coordinative flexibility, but only in the MIP task, while acknowledging that these findings are not accompanied by direct fall-related outcomes. In this context, greater movement complexity can be framed as a property that may support a wider repertoire of responses under perturbation; however, implications for fall prevention should be considered tentative and hypothesis-generating only. Therefore, the simultaneous upward trends in MIE and LyEM, despite non-significance, are best interpreted as preliminary indicators of more adaptable patterns, warranting confirmation in studies incorporating overground walking and fall-related endpoints. Taken together, any directional inferences from LyEM/MIE should be made with caution, as similar numerical changes can arise from distinct mechanisms (e.g., adaptive reorganization vs. increased signal noise). Future work should triangulate these nonlinear measures with overground walking, more clinical balance tests, and fall outcomes to determine whether the observed patterns reflect functionally meaningful adaptation.

It is important to note that, in addition to the small sample size, participants were institutionalized and highly frail, which limited the intensity of the exercise sessions. Completing only three sessions of predominantly low-intensity exercise per week may not have been sufficient to generate significant changes. The reduced sample size limits the analyses' statistical power, increasing the likelihood of Type II error and may partially explain the absence of statistically significant results. Therefore, future studies are encouraged to adopt more regular weekly practice, ideally on a daily basis, to increase potential adaptations and benefits. Although marching-in-place is less ecologically valid than overground walking, its use provided a safe and standardized dynamic task compatible with non-linear analysis in this single-institution, frail cohort. Future studies should complement this approach with overground walking under controlled linear paths to enhance ecological validity while preserving analytical consistency.

Given the quasi-experimental pre–post design without a control group, the internal validity of the study is limited. Potential influences such as learning effects, natural day-to-day variability, fluctuations in health status or medication, and regression to the mean cannot be excluded. The absence of a control group limits the interpretation of the data, especially because no reference values for these tests and for the nonlinear (innovative) methodologies that were applied. It is recommended that future studies include two control groups: one composed of frail older adults who do not carry out the exercise program, as this group would make it possible to confirm that the changes, i.e., the possible improvements observed, are indeed the result of the program; and a second control group composed of non-frail and physically active older adults. Comparing the results and improvements observed in the frail group with those of non-frail, active older adults would make it possible to determine whether the changes approach the performance levels expected in healthier and more physically active older populations. Generalizability is limited to similar institutionalized, frail cohorts under supervised low-to-moderate-intensity programs. Future research should also explore the optimal duration and intensity of such exercise programs in order to maximize health and functional benefits for older adults.

5. Conclusions

This exploratory study did not detect statistically significant pre- to post-intervention changes in non-linear motor coordination metrics; however, small-to-moderate effect sizes, particularly during marching in place, suggest trends compatible with increased motor complexity and adaptability following participation in MIND&GAIT. These patterns should be interpreted as preliminary and hypothesis-generating, rather than as evidence of

https://doi.org/10.3390/healthcare14060770

confirmed functional benefits. In line with the study design, sample size and frailty profile, no causal inferences can be drawn.

Regarding potential implications for stability and fall risk, the observed changes in LyEM and MIE may be consistent with mechanisms underpinning more flexible and adaptive coordination; nevertheless, such interpretations remain tentative, as no direct fall-related outcomes were assessed. Future research with larger samples, controlled overground walking protocols, appropriate control groups, and fall-relevant endpoints (e.g., prospective fall incidence or validated clinical proxies) is needed to verify whether these biomechanical trends translate into clinically meaningful improvements.

Taken together, the present findings highlight the feasibility of applying non-linear analyses with wearable sensors in institutionalized, frail older adults and motivate further investigation. Until corroborated by adequately powered trials, the effects observed here should be viewed as initial signals that warrant confirmation, rather than as definitive evidence of intervention efficacy.

Author Contributions: Conceptualization, resources, C.M., F.R. and M.B.; methodology, funding acquisition, C.M., F.R., D.C. and M.B.; software, M.B.; validation, data curation, C.M., S.A., F.R. and M.B.; formal analysis, C.M. and M.B.; investigation, S.A.; writing—original draft preparation, C.M. and S.A.; writing—review and editing, visualization, C.M., S.A., F.R., D.C. and M.B.; supervision, C.M. and F.R.; project administration, C.M. All authors have read and agreed to the published version of the manuscript.

Funding: The researchers are supported by the Portuguese Foundation for Science and Technology, I.P., by means of SPRINT—Sport Physical activity and Health Research & Innovation Center [UID/06185/2025][UID/PRR/06185/2025][UID/PRR2/06185/2025], and Life Quality Research Center (LQRC), Santarém, Portugal, grant number UID/CED/04748/2023. This study is part of the MIND&GAIT project (POCI-01-0145-FEDER-023822) which was funded by COMPETE2020 program, Portugal. João Apóstolo was the PI of the project. Rita Santos-Rocha and Fátima Ramalho were the Pis and creators of the exercise program. The funders had no role in the design of the study; in the collection, analyses, or interpretation of data; in the writing of the manuscript, or in the decision to publish the results.

Institutional Review Board Statement: The study was conducted in accordance with the Declaration of Helsinki and approved by the Institutional Ethics Committee of Polytechnic Institute of Santarém (approval number 10-2024 ESDRM, approval date 25 March 2024).

Informed Consent Statement: Informed consent was obtained from all subjects involved in the study.

Data Availability Statement: The data are not publicly available due to ethical restrictions. However, portions of the dataset may be made available upon reasonable request and subject to approval by the institutional ethics committee. The ethics committee only authorized data sharing among the researchers responsible for the study.

Acknowledgments: During the preparation of this manuscript, the authors used M365 Copilot to assist with translation tasks and to refine the writing of small sections of the text. After using this tool, all content was thoroughly reviewed, edited, and validated by the authors, who take full responsibility for the final version of the manuscript.

Conflicts of Interest: The authors declare no conflicts of interest.

Abbreviations

The following abbreviations are used in this manuscript:

 https://doi.org/10.3390/healthcare14060770

ADLs	Activities of Daily Life
FFT	Fast Fourier Transform
FNN	False-Nearest-Neighbors
HR	Heart Rate
IMU/IMUs	Inertial Measurement Unit(s)
LyE	Lyapunov Exponent
LyEM	Multivariate Lyapunov Exponent
MIE	Multivariate Incremental Entropy
MIP	Marching in place
PE	Directory of open access journals
PE	Physical Exercise
RPE	Rating of Perceived Exertion (Modified Borg)
STROBE	Strengthening the Reporting of Observational Studies in Epidemiology
STS	Sit-to-Stand
TREND	Transparent Reporting of Evaluations with Nonrandomized Designs
1RM	One-Repetition Maximum
3D	Three-Dimensional

References

1. Colón-Emeric, C.; McDermott, C.; Lee, D.; Berry, S. Risk Assessment and Prevention of Falls in Older Community-Dwelling Adults: A Review. *JAMA* **2024**, *331*, 1397–1406. [CrossRef]
2. Afiah, I.N.; Nakashima, H.; Loh, P.Y.; Muraki, S. An exploratory investigation of changes in gait parameters with age in elderly Japanese women. *SpringerPlus* **2016**, *5*, 1069. [CrossRef]
3. Gabriel, G.; Harris, L.; Gnanasegaram, J.; Cushing, S.; Gordon, K.; Haycock, B.; Campos, J. Age-related changes to vestibular heave and pitch perception and associations with postural control. *Sci. Rep.* **2022**, *12*, 6426. [CrossRef] [PubMed]
4. Hollman, J.; McDade, E.; Petersen, R. Normative spatiotemporal gait parameters in older adults. *Gait Posture* **2011**, *34*, 111–118. [CrossRef]
5. Du, S.; Ma, X.; Wang, J.; Mi, Y.; Zhang, J.; Du, C.; Li, X.; Tan, H.; Liang, C.; Yang, T.; et al. Spatiotemporal gait parameter fluctuations in older adults affected by mild cognitive impairment: Comparisons among three cognitive dual-task tests. *BMC Geriatr.* **2023**, *23*, 603. [CrossRef]
6. Sadeh, S.; Gobert, D.; Shen, K.-H.; Foroughi, F.; Hsiao, H. Biomechanical and neuromuscular control characteristics of sit-to-stand transfer in young and older adults: A systematic review with implications for balance regulation mechanisms. *Clin. Biomech.* **2023**, *109*, 106068. [CrossRef]
7. Ramalho, F.; Santos-Rocha, R.; Branco, M.; Moniz-Pereira, V.; André, H.-I.; Veloso, A.; Carnide, F. Effect of 6-month community-based exercise interventions on gait and functional fitness of an older population: A quasi-experimental study. *Clin. Interv. Aging* **2018**, *13*, 595–606. [CrossRef]
8. Zhang, S.-K.; Qian, G.; Xu, H.; Gu, M.-L.; Mao, S.-J.; Wang, Y.; Zhang, Y.; Zhou, W. Effects of different exercise modalities on balance performance in healthy older adults: A systematic review and network meta-analysis of randomized controlled trials. *BMC Geriatr.* **2025**, *25*, 570. [CrossRef]
9. Camomilla, V.; Bergamini, E.; Fantozzi, S.; Vannozzi, G. Trends Supporting the In-Field Use of Wearable Inertial Sensors for Sport Performance Evaluation: A Systematic Review. *Sensors* **2018**, *18*, 873. [CrossRef] [PubMed]
10. Kędziorek, J.; Błażkiewicz, M. Nonlinear Measures to Evaluate Upright Postural Stability: A Systematic Review. *Entropy* **2020**, *22*, 1357. [CrossRef]
11. Brígida, N.; Catela, D.; Mercê, C.; Branco, M. Predictability and Complexity of Fine and Gross Motor Skills in Fibromyalgia Patients: A Pilot Study. *Sports* **2024**, *12*, 90. [CrossRef]
12. Yentes, J.M.; Raffalt, P.C. Entropy Analysis in Gait Research: Methodological Considerations and Recommendations. *Ann. Biomed. Eng.* **2021**, *49*, 979–990. [CrossRef] [PubMed]
13. Lipsitz, L.A.; Goldberger, A.L. Loss of 'complexity' and aging. Potential applications of fractals and chaos theory to senescence. *JAMA* **1992**, *267*, 1806–1809. [CrossRef]
14. Blons, E.; Arsac, L.; Gilfriche, P.; Deschodt-Arsac, V. Multiscale Entropy of Cardiac and Postural Control Reflects a Flexible Adaptation to a Cognitive Task. *Entropy* **2019**, *21*, 1024. [CrossRef]
15. Mercê, C.; Davids, K.; Cordovil, R.; Catela, D.; Branco, M. Learning to Cycle: Why Is the Balance Bike More Efficient than the Bicycle with Training Wheels? The Lyapunov's Answer. *J. Funct. Morphol. Kinesiol.* **2024**, *9*, 266. [CrossRef] [PubMed]

https://doi.org/10.3390/healthcare14060770

16. Winter, L.; Taylor, P.; Bellenger, C.; Grimshaw, P.; Crowther, R. The application of the Lyapunov Exponent to analyse human performance: A systematic review. *J. Sports Sci.* **2023**, *41*, 1994–2013. [CrossRef]
17. Mehdizadeh, S. The largest Lyapunov exponent of gait in young and elderly individuals: A systematic review. *Gait Posture* **2018**, *60*, 241–250. [CrossRef]
18. Promsri, A.; Cholamjiak, P.; Federolf, P. Walking Stability and Risk of Falls. *Bioengineering* **2023**, *10*, 471. [CrossRef]
19. Santos-Rocha, R.; Freitas, J.; Ramalho, F.; Pimenta, N.; Costa Couto, F.; Apóstolo, J. Development and validation of a complex intervention: A physical exercise programme aimed at delaying the functional decline in frail older adults. *Nurs. Open* **2020**, *7*, 274–284. [CrossRef] [PubMed]
20. Rikli, R.E.; Jones, C.J. Development and Validation of Criterion-Referenced Clinically Relevant Fitness Standards for Maintaining Physical Independence in Later Years. *Gerontol.* **2012**, *53*, 255–267. [CrossRef]
21. The MathWorks, Inc. *MATLAB (Version R2025a)*; The MathWorks, Inc.: Natick, MA, USA, 2025.
22. Crenna, F.; Rossi, G.B.; Berardengo, M. Filtering Biomechanical Signals in Movement Analysis. *Sensors* **2021**, *21*, 4580. [CrossRef] [PubMed]
23. Gustafsson, F. Determining the initial states in forward-backward filtering. *IEEE Trans. Signal Process.* **1996**, *44*, 988–992. [CrossRef]
24. Takens, F. Detecting strange attractors in turbulence. In *Dynamical Systems and Turbulence, Warwick 1980*; Springer: Berlin/Heidelberg, Germany, 1981; pp. 366–381.
25. Hegger, R.; Kantz, H.; Schreiber, T. Practical implementation of nonlinear time series methods: The TISEAN package. *Chaos Interdiscip. J. Nonlinear Sci.* **1999**, *9*, 413–435. [CrossRef] [PubMed]
26. Wolf, A.; Swift, J.B.; Swinney, H.L.; Vastano, J.A. Determining Lyapunov exponents from a time series. *Phys. D Nonlinear Phenom.* **1985**, *16*, 285–317. [CrossRef]
27. Cohen, J. *Statistical Power Analysis for the Behavioral Sciences*, 2nd ed.; Lawrence Erlbaum Associates: Mahwah, NJ, USA, 1988.
28. Hu, Q.; Chen, X.; Luo, S.; Wang, Y.; Fan, P.; Wu, X.; Zhou, H.; Xu, H.; Li, N.; Cai, X. Phase angle as a predictor of motor function decline in children with Duchenne muscular dystrophy. *BMC Pediatr.* **2025**, *25*, 488. [CrossRef]
29. Huang, Q.; Liu, H.; Chien, C.-W. Intra-limb joint coordination measures of upper limb and hand movements: A systematic review. *Gait Posture* **2023**, *108*, 289–300. [CrossRef]
30. Raffalt, P.C.; Senderling, B.; Stergiou, N. Filtering affects the calculation of the largest Lyapunov exponent. *Comput. Biol. Med.* **2020**, *122*, 103786. [CrossRef] [PubMed]
31. Amirpourabasi, A.; Lamb, S.; Chow, J.; Williams, G. Nonlinear Dynamic Measures of Walking in Healthy Older Adults: A Systematic Scoping Review. *Sensors* **2022**, *22*, 4408. [CrossRef]
32. Mao, Q.; Zheng, W.; Shi, M.; Yang, F. Scientometric Research and Critical Analysis of Gait and Balance in Older Adults. *Sensors* **2024**, *24*, 3199. [CrossRef]
33. Mercê, C.; Sousa, M.; Bernardino, S.; Saramago, N.; Pereira, H.; Santos-Rocha, R. Efectos de intervenciones basadas en el modelo transteórico para incrementar la actividad física en adultos mayores: Revisión sistemática. *Retos* **2025**, *68*, 1997–2007. [CrossRef]
34. Charal, C.M.S.; Westphal, G.; Faúndez-Casanova, C.; Castilho, M.M.; Amaral, M.F.; Soares, G.S.; Martins, F.M.; Borim, M.L.C.; Candido, I.C. Motor coordination: Quality of elderly movement. *Res. Soc. Dev.* **2022**, *11*, e28111629255. [CrossRef]
35. Dunsky, A. The Effect of Balance and Coordination Exercises on Quality of Life in Older Adults: A Mini-Review. *Front. Aging Neurosci.* **2019**, *11*, 318. [CrossRef]
36. Wang, J.; Li, Y.; Yang, G.-Y.; Jin, K. Age-Related Dysfunction in Balance: A Comprehensive Review of Causes, Consequences, and Interventions. *Aging Dis.* **2024**, *16*, 714–737. [CrossRef] [PubMed]
37. Huang, Y.; Zhao, Y. Efficacy of Exercise on Muscle Function and Physical Performance in Older Adults with Sarcopenia: An Updated Systematic Review and Meta-Analysis. *Int. J. Environ. Res. Public Health* **2022**, *19*, 8212. [CrossRef]
38. Stergiou, N.; Decker, L.M. Human movement variability, nonlinear dynamics, and pathology: Is there a connection? *Hum. Mov. Sci.* **2011**, *30*, 869–888. [CrossRef] [PubMed]
39. Stergiou, N.; Harbourne, R.; Cavanaugh, J. Optimal movement variability: A new theoretical perspective for neurologic physical therapy. *J. Neurol. Phys. Ther.* **2006**, *30*, 120–129. [CrossRef] [PubMed]
40. Busa, M.A.; van Emmerik, R.E.A. Multiscale entropy: A tool for understanding the complexity of postural control. *J. Sport Health Sci.* **2016**, *5*, 44–51. [CrossRef]

healthcare

MDPI

Article

Comparison of Strength Training Interventions on Functional Performance in Frail Nursing Home Residents

Helena Vila [1], Carmen Ferragut [2,*], Luis Javier Chirosa [3], Virginia Serrano-Gómez [1,*], Óscar García-García [1], Daniel Jerez-Mayorga [3,4], Ángela Rodríguez-Perea [3,5] and José María Cancela [1]

1 Department of Specific Didactics, Faculty of Education and Sport Sciences, University of Vigo, 36005 Pontevedra, Spain; evila@uvigo.es (H.V.); oscargarcia@uvigo.es (Ó.G.-G.)
2 Area of Physical and Sports Education, Faculty of Medicine and Health Sciences, Department of Biomedical Sciences, University of Alcalá, 28801 Madrid, Spain
3 Department of Physical Education and Sports, Faculty of Sport Sciences, Sport and Health University Research Institute (iMUDS), University of Granada, 18071 Granada, Spain; lchirosa@ugr.es (L.J.C.); djerezmayorga@ugr.es (D.J.-M.); arodrp@unileon.es (Á.R.-P.)
4 Exercise and Rehabilitation Sciences Institute, Faculty of Rehabilitation Sciences, Universidad Andres Bello, Santiago 7591538, Chile
5 Faculty of Physical Activity and Sports Sciences, Department of Physical Education and Sport, Universidad de León, 24007 León, Spain
* Correspondence: carmen.ferragut@uah.es (C.F.); vserrano@uvigo.es (V.S.-G.)

Abstract

Background/Objectives: Frailty and functional decline represent major challenges for aging populations, particularly among institutionalized older adults. Preserving functional capacity is essential to maintain autonomy, mobility, and quality of life. This study aimed to compare the effects of two strength training interventions—functional electromechanical dynamometer (FEMD) training and weighted vest training—on peak concentric and eccentric force during the sit-to-stand task, as well as on functional performance and body composition in frail nursing home residents. **Methods:** A pilot quasi-experimental study with a non-randomized control group was conducted in 19 older adults (mean age: 86.3 ± 5.8 years). Participants were allocated to FEMD training (EG1, n = 6), weighted vest training (EG2, n = 6), or a control group (CG, n = 7). Training was performed twice weekly for eight weeks. Assessments included body composition, handgrip strength, 30 s chair stand test, 3 m walking speed, and peak concentric and eccentric force during the sit-to-stand movement. Data were analyzed using mixed-model ANOVA and complementary within-group analyses. **Results:** No significant group × moment interactions were observed. However, EG1 demonstrated significant within-group improvements in chair stand performance (+4.8 repetitions, $p = 0.006$), walking speed (+0.1 $m \cdot s^{-1}$, $p = 0.030$), concentric peak force (+46.5%, $p = 0.008$), and eccentric peak force (+34%, $p = 0.047$). EG2 showed a smaller but significant increase in eccentric peak force (+6.1%, $p = 0.019$), without functional improvements. Body composition changes were modest, with EG1 showing increases in weight and BMI without concomitant fat mass gains. **Conclusions:** In this pilot quasi-experimental study, functional electromechanical dynamometer-based training was associated with improvements in neuromuscular performance, particularly concentric peak force. However, no significant group × moment interactions were observed, indicating that differential effects between interventions cannot be established. Functional improvements should be interpreted cautiously. The present results should therefore be considered exploratory and hypothesis-generating. These findings suggest that FEMD-based training may be a feasible and potentially beneficial functional strength training strategy for frail institutionalized older adults, which should be confirmed in adequately powered randomized controlled trials.

Healthcare **2026**, *14*, 303

https://doi.org/10.3390/healthcare14030303

Keywords: strength training; physical performance; frailty; quality of life; functional electromechanical dynamometer

1. Introduction

As global populations continue to age, the prevalence of frailty and functional decline among older adults has become a significant public health concern [1]. Sedentary life-styles, often intensified by institutional living environments, accelerate the deterioration of physical function, increase the risk of falls, and reduce quality of life [1]. Frailty, characterized by decreased physiological resilience, makes older adults particularly vulnerable to functional loss, disability, and dependency. Consequently, interventions that counteract frailty by improving muscle strength and motor control are essential for sustaining health and delaying functional deterioration.

Walking speed is a critical indicator of health and functionality in older adults, as it is directly associated with morbidity and mortality [2]. Gait speed has been proposed as a reliable proxy for frailty status and a predictor of adverse health outcomes, including hospitalization and mortality [3,4]. Reduced walking speed is linked to higher risk of falls and loss of independence [5], highlighting the importance of maintaining functional capacity to preserve quality of life [6]. Since walking speed depends on muscle strength and endurance, engaging in strength exercises and mobility-enhancing activities can mitigate age-related declines and improve quality of life [7,8].

Strength training has emerged as a fundamental strategy for preventing and counteracting frailty in older adults [9]. Evidence consistently highlights the benefits of resistance training for improving muscle strength, mass, and overall functional capacity [7,10,11]. Furthermore, this type of exercise is recognized as an evidence-based intervention to delay frailty progression, enhance independence, and improve multidimensional health outcomes, including mental well-being and self-perceived quality of life.

Despite these benefits, there remains a need for effective and adaptable exercise protocols that can be safely implemented in institutional settings. Electromechanical and weighted strength training methods offer practical and individualized approaches to enhance physical and functional capacities in frail older populations. By focusing on frail institutionalized adults, this research explores how these training modalities contribute to maintaining independence and overall health status, addressing critical aspects of frailty management and quality of life.

The eccentric phase of muscle contraction, during which muscles lengthen under tension, has garnered attention for its unique advantages [12]. For example, programs combining strength and balance training have been shown to increase walking speed, thereby improving mobility and reducing fall risk in older adults [13].

Traditional methods such as free weights [14] and resistance machines [15] require engagement of both concentric and eccentric phases. The concentric phase occurs when the muscle shortens to produce external work, while the eccentric phase involves muscle lengthening, generating both positive and negative work [16].

New technologies, such as Functional Electromechanical Dynamometry (FEMD), represent advanced methodological approaches for quantifying neuromuscular performance variables—specifically strength, power, and velocity—during functional tasks [17]. Compared to traditional isokinetic or handheld dynamometry, FEMD offers superior ecological validity by replicating real-life or sport-specific motor actions [17,18].

The eccentric phase allows training with heavier loads—20% to 50% greater than the concentric contractions [19]. Strength gains from eccentric training are often superior to

 https://doi.org/10.3390/healthcare14030303

conventional methods [20]. Additionally, eccentric exercise improves muscle and joint flexibility by increasing the extensibility of fibers and connective tissue, thereby reducing injury risk, optimizing range of motion, and enhancing walking speed [21,22]. Studies show that eccentric contractions generate greater muscular forces with lower energy costs [23,24], which is particularly advantageous for older adults experiencing declines in muscle mass and metabolic efficiency [24]. Eccentric training also promotes neuromuscular adaptations such as improved intermuscular coordination and greater motor unit activation, both critical for motor control, stability, and fall prevention [25,26]. High-intensity eccentric contractions accelerate strength gains and hypertrophy, directly contributing to improvements in walking speed [24].

Although eccentric training can initially cause acute muscle damage and delayed onset muscle soreness (DOMS), these responses are part of the adaptation process and diminish with progressive training [27]. This phenomenon, known as the "repeated bout effect", reduces susceptibility to muscle damage over time, allowing long-term benefits to outweigh the initial discomfort [27].

Given this evidence, eccentric training appears to be an effective strategy for optimizing physical performance, improving metabolic and cardiovascular health, and preventing injuries in older adults. Therefore, this study aimed to compare the effects of two strength interventions—functional electromechanical dynamometer training and weighted training—on peak force during concentric and eccentric phases of the sit-to-stand movement in older adults residing in a nursing home. Additionally, we evaluated the impact of both interventions on functional capacity (gait speed, hand-grip strength, and sit-to-stand performance) and body composition. We hypothesized that eccentric-focused strength training would lead to greater improvements in peak force compared to traditional combined concentric-eccentric training.

We hypothesized that strength training performed with a functional electromechanical dynamometry would lead to greater improvements in peak force compared to similar exercises performed with a weighted vest.

2. Materials and Methods

2.1. Participants

Of the 22 older adults initially recruited, 19 completed the study. Three participants voluntarily withdrew due to reasons such as leaving the residence or experiencing physical discomfort, resulting in a final sample of 19 individuals (age: 86.3 ± 5.8 years; sex (female/male): 12/7). Participants were assigned to one of three groups: Group 1 (EG1, n = 6), which performed strength training using FEMD; Group 2 (EG2, n = 6) which trained with weighted vests; and a Control Group (CG, n = 7), which received no intervention (e.g., "continued with their usual daily activities and standard nursing home care"). Regarding group allocation, a participant-preference quasi-experimental design was used [28]. The control group consisted of individuals who chose not to participate in either of the two training programs. The two experimental groups were assigned by the facility's physiotherapist based on organizational criteria. Importantly, the research team did not participate in the allocation process at any point. Inclusion criteria included the ability to perform the exercises proposed in the intervention and the ability to attend 85% of the sessions. Exclusion criteria included any condition that contraindicated strength training, difficulty following the instructor's instructions, or expressing a desire to withdraw from the program. Procedures, potential risks or discomfort associated with the experiments were explained to participants, who then gave their written informed consent. The study design and protocol adhered to the tenets of the Declaration of Helsinki and was approved by the University Review Board (CEIC-14-1009-17). The sample size calculation revealed

https://doi.org/10.3390/healthcare14030303

that 18 participants [29,30] were estimated to be sufficient for this study to detect an effect size of 0.7 ($\alpha = 0.05$; $1 - \beta = 0.90$) (G*power V3.1, Dusseldorf University, Germany). Based on this estimation, the study was designed with three conditions, allocating six participants to each group (n = 6). This distribution was considered appropriate given the expected large effect size, the use of repeated measures to enhance statistical sensitivity, and practical constraints related to participant recruitment in this specific population. Such an approach ensures methodological rigor while maintaining feasibility in a controlled experimental setting.

2.2. Experimental Design and Protocol

A pilot quasi-experimental study with a non-randomized control group was conducted to compare the effects of two strength training interventions (FEMD and weighted vest training) on execution speed and peak force during the concentric and eccentric phases of the sit-to-stand movement.

Baseline and post-intervention assessments were carried out over two no-consecutive days each, due to the number of participants. Height was measured first, followed by body composition. Subsequently, the hand grip strength test was performed, along with the 30 s sit-to-stand test and a 3 m walking speed test. On the first day, participants underwent a familiarization session with the FEMD, performing four sets of six repetitions. On the second day, the sit-to-stand test was performed using the FEMD, with a 48 h rest period between pre- and post-intervention assessments. A 48 h interval was selected to ensure adequate recovery and to minimize potential fatigue or acute learning effects associated with the familiarization protocol. Additionally, prior research using electromechanical dynamometry and sit-to-stand testing in older adults has employed rest periods of 24–48 h between familiarization and baseline testing without adverse effects on test reliability or performance outcomes [17,31,32]. Based on this evidence, we consider the 48 h interval sufficient to prevent residual fatigue while preserving the intended benefits of familiarization.

The intervention lasted for two months, with a frequency of two sessions per week (Tuesdays and Thursdays), with sessions lasting approximately 45–60 min (Figure 1).

The training consisted of five lower-body exercises and three upper-body exercises. Participants performed four sets of six repetitions for each exercise, with a three-minute rest between sets. They were encouraged to perform the downward (eccentric) phase of each movement in a controlled manner. The total training volume (sets × repetitions × load) was equally distributed across the intervention groups.

All participants began the training with an initial load of 3 kg. When participants were able to complete the prescribed sets and repetitions while maintaining the required intensity and recovering adequately between sessions, the load was increased by 0.5, 1, 1.5, or 2 kg in the following session, based on individual performance. This progression protocol was applied equally in both intervention groups. Participants had to stand up as quickly as possible and sit down slowly. When each subject completed the sets and repetitions while maintaining the required intensity and adequately recovering in each session. This series-by-series progression strategy has been shown to be effective in promoting rapid strength gains in previous short-term studies [33–35]. Participants were instructed to inform their trainers if they experienced any discomfort during the training. Regarding perceived effort, the use of the Borg Rating of Perceived Exertion Scale was excluded, as many participants presented cognitive impairment or dementia, which could compromise the reliability of self-reported exercise intensity [36,37].

https://doi.org/10.3390/healthcare14030303

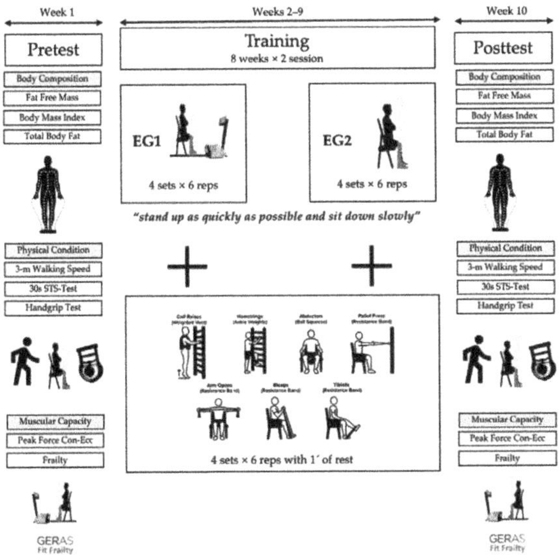

Figure 1. Strength training program.

Partial Blinding of Assessors

In our study, strength assessment using dynamometry was conducted by a researcher who did not participate in the training sessions, acting as a blinded evaluator for both the pre- and post-intervention measurements. This approach minimizes the risk of bias in this key variable. Previous studies employing blinded evaluator designs have been considered methodologically robust in interventions with older adults [38,39]. The other functional tests (chair-stand, gait speed, etc.) were performed by other team members, including the trainers. Although these evaluators were not blinded to group allocation, all tests followed standardized and objective protocols (repetitions, times, distances), thereby reducing the likelihood of measurement bias.

2.3. Experimental Protocol

2.3.1. Body Composition and Physical Activity Habits

A basic anthropometric assessment of weight and height was conducted, as well as the Body Mass Index (BMI). The anthropometric measurements followed the protocols of the International Society for the advancement of Kinanthropometry (ISAK) [40]. Height was measured with participants standing barefoot using a portable stadiometer (Seca GmbH & Co., KG, Hamburg, Germany) with an accuracy of 0.1 cm. Weight and body composition was assessed using bioelectrical impedance analysis (BIA) with participants standing, without shoes or socks, using a Tanita MC-780 multifrequency segmental body composition analyzer (Amsterdam, The Netherlands) with an accuracy of 0.1 kg.

The variables obtained from BIA included fat mass (FM), fat-free mass (FFM), total body water (TBW), visceral fat index, daily caloric intake (DCI), and basal metabolic rate (BMR). BMI was calculated by dividing body weight (kg) by height squared (m^2). This BIA technology has been recently validated in adults with varying levels of physical activity [41]. Visceral fat was indirectly estimated and expressed using a specific rating scale ranging from 0 to 59 arbitrary units (AU), where values from 1 to 12 indicate a healthy level of visceral fat, and values from 13 to 59 indicate excess visceral fat [42].

Therefore, the Physical Activity Scale for the Elderly (PASE) was administered to collect data on physical activity, household tasks, and occupational activities performed

https://doi.org/10.3390/healthcare14030303

over the previous seven days. This scale was specifically developed to assess physical activity levels in epidemiological studies involving individuals aged 65 years and older. In addition, PASE scores are commonly used as part of frailty assessment protocols, as reduced physical activity is a key component of the frailty phenotype [43]. In this study, the PASE was used to characterize baseline physical activity levels and to complement frailty assessment, providing contextual information about participants' activity habits.

2.3.2. Handgrip Test

Handgrip strength (HG) was measured using a Jamar hand dynamometer (Sammons Preston Inc., Bolingbrook, IL, USA). Participants were instructed to stand and hold the dynamometer with their arm parallel to their body, ensuring it was not pressed against their body. Both hands were tested during this assessment. The width of the handle was adjusted to fit each participant's hand, ensuring that the middle phalanx rested comfortably on the inner handle. Participants were allowed one practice trial, followed by three test trials, with the best score used for analysis. HG was expressed in kilograms (kg). Testing was conducted on both arms. A manual muscle strength of 30 kg or greater for men and 20 kg or greater for women was considered normal; values below these thresholds were deemed inadequate [44,45].

2.3.3. Chair Stand Test

The participant begins seated in the middle of the chair, with their back straight, feet flat on the floor, and arms crossed over their chest. At the "go" signal, the participant should stand up completely and return to the initial position as many times as possible within 30 s. It is recommended to demonstrate the exercise slowly first, allowing the participant to observe the correct execution, followed by a faster demonstration for better understanding. Before starting the test, the participant should perform the exercise one or two times to ensure correct execution [46].

2.3.4. Walking 3 Meter Speed

The walking speed over three meters was evaluated by timing how long each participant took to cover the distance [47]. Participants started behind a marked line, and at the signal, the stopwatch was activated as they began to walk. The stopwatch was stopped when the participant crossed the finish line with their last foot, both of which were marked on the ground. Two attempts were conducted, and the time from the best attempt was recorded and converted to meters per second for analysis, with a rest period of three minutes between repetitions.

2.3.5. Strength Measurement

Participants sat on a firm, upright chair (measuring 40 cm in height) with their arms crossed, and their hip, knee, and ankle joints were positioned at roughly 90 degrees. Following the countdown of 3, 2, 1, participants were instructed to initiate the concentric phase at maximum velocity upon command from this position. Concentric and eccentric peak force was measured using a sit-to-stand test with 5 repetitions on the FEMD (Myoquality M1, Myoquality Solutions, Granada, Spain [17,48]. The weight set to complete the set was 3 kg. The FEMD was set up in 'Tonic Mode', which featured an external load designed to mimic a free weight.

The linear displacement of each participant was measured while standing, using a FEMD rope attached to a harness secured to their waistcoat. The maximum force in kilograms for each repetition was captured during both the concentric and eccentric phases via the FEMD software Myosoft 2.8.4. The test was considered reliable if the knees and trunk were fully extended at the conclusion of the concentric phase [17].

 https://doi.org/10.3390/healthcare14030303

Both muscular strength and power were determined using a FEMD (Myoquality M1, Myoquality Solutions, Granada, Spain). The peak concentric and eccentric force during the sit-to-stand movement was measured, using a reliable instrument for squat protocols, allowing for the reliable evaluation of these parameters [31]. The operation of the FEMD for obtaining these variables involves the performer applying forces to a rope wound around a roller, controlling and measuring both force and linear velocity [18]. A load cell detects the tension applied to the rope, and the resulting signal is converted from analog to digital with a resolution of 12 bits. Speed and displacement data are obtained using a 2500 ppr encoder coupled to the roller. The sensors collect various data at a frequency of 1 kHz [31].

2.4. Statistical Analysis

Statistical analyses were conducted using SPSS (Version 29.0; IBM Corp., Armonk, NY, USA). Descriptive statistics were reported as means and standard deviations (SD) for continuous variables and percentages for categorical variables. Pre-intervention differences among the three groups (EG1, EG2, CG) were examined using paired-sample t tests or analysis of variance (ANOVA). The Shapiro–Wilk test was applied to assess the normality of continuous dependent variables across groups.

A mixed-model ANOVA, which integrates between-subject and within-subject factors, was employed to evaluate interaction effects between moment (pre vs. post) and group (EG1, EG2, CG). This approach is widely recognized as standard practice for assessing intervention effects in exercise physiology [49]. Compared to the general linear model, mixed models offer superior handling of missing data in repeated-measures designs [50]. Accordingly, mixed-model ANOVA was used to estimate intervention effects based on significant moment × group interactions. Analyses adhered to the intent-to-treat principle.

Graphical representations (Figure 2) illustrate the relationship between 3 m walking speed (m/s) and eccentric peak force (kg) at pre- and post-intervention across experimental groups. Statistical significance was set at $p < 0.05$ (two-tailed). Post hoc comparisons were conducted using the Bonferroni adjustment.

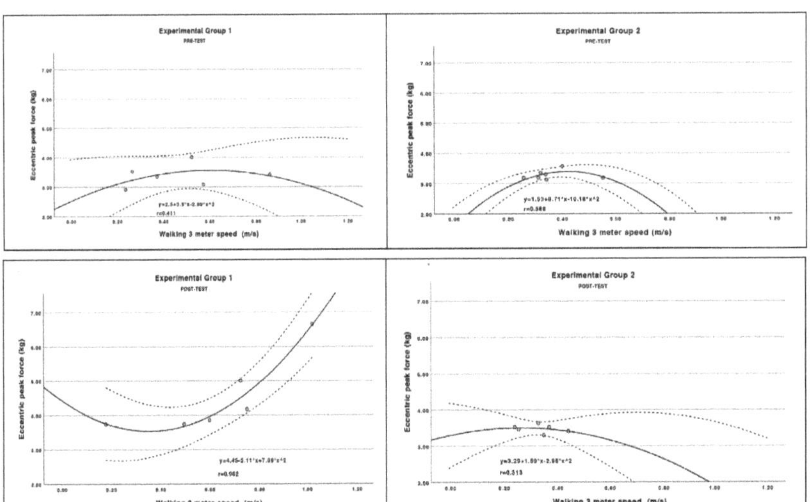

Figure 2. Correlations between peak eccentric force and walking speed in both strength intervention groups during the pre-test and post-test.

https://doi.org/10.3390/healthcare14030303

3. Results

3.1. Physical Characteristics of the Sample

The physical characteristics of the sample are presented in Table 1. The results for the three groups (EG1, CC, and EG2) before and after the intervention are detailed in Table 2, focusing on variables related to body composition, physical condition, and muscular strength.

Table 1. Descriptive analysis of the body composition in older adults organized by groups.

	All (n = 19)	CG (n = 7)	EG1 (n = 6)	EG2 (n = 6)
	Mean ± SD	Mean ± SD	Mean ± SD	Mean ± SD
Age (years)	86.7 ± 5.8	86.2 ± 7.8	86.2 ± 5.9	87.4 ± 4.3
Weight (kg)	64.1 ± 10.6	68.3 ± 15.4	62.8 ± 9.4	61.6 ± 6.4
Height (cm)	153.6 ± 6.8	154.9 ± 7.4	152.0 ± 6.3	153.9 ± 7.5
Waist Hip Ratio	0.9 ± 0.1	0.96 ± 0.0	0.9 ± 0.1	0.9 ± 0.0
Sex, female (%)	63.1	71.4	66.70	50.0

Legend: CG = Control Group; EG1 = Experimental group with dynamometer; EG2 = Experimental group with weighted vest.

Table 2. Performance Changes in Training and Control Groups Following 8-Week Intervention in Dwelling Older Adults (Mixed ANOVA 2 × 3).

	Control Group (CG)		Experimental Group 1 (EG1)		Experimental Group 2 (EG2)		ANOVA MIXED (2 × 3)		
	Pre Mean ± SD	Post Mean ± SD	Pre Mean ± SD	Post Mean ± SD	Pre Mean ± SD	Post Mean ± SD	Group Sig	Moment Sig	Group × Moment Sig
Body Composition									
Fat-Free Mass (kg)	50.0 ± 4.4	47.6 ± 6.4	40.9 ± 5.8	42.9 ± 6.0 *	38.9 ± 7.5	39.7 ± 8.6	0.192	0.443	0.843
BMI (kg/m^2)	29.2 ± 8.3	33.2 ± 13.1	27.1 ± 2.8	28.3 ± 3.6 *	26.1 ± 2.3	26.6 ± 2.8	0.569	0.435	0.759
Total Body Fat (kg)	22.6 ± 14.6	25.9 ± 17.9	22.5 ± 2.7	20.6 ± 7.5	19.7 ± 6.1	20.9 ± 5.5 *	0.468	0.205	0.512
Body Water (kg)	33.4 ± 4.6	35.5 ± 5.5	30.0 ± 4.0	30.7 ± 4.5	28.2 ± 5.2	29.1 ± 4.9	0.116	0.387	0.780
Visceral Fat Indicator	16.2 ± 4.7	18.3 ± 3.1	13.0 ± 4.7	12.8 ± 4.3	12.7 ± 2.1	13.8 ± 2.6	0.790	0.998	0.917
DCI/BMR (kcal)	1421.6 ± 165.1	1512.3 ± 167.7	1282.5 ± 154.6	1295.4 ± 172.8 *	1206.7 ± 172.4	1257.5 ± 178.0	0.175	0.548	0.895
Physical Condition									
3 m Walking speed (m/s)	0.5 ± 0.1	0.4 ± 0.1	0.5 ± 0.2	0.6 ± 0.3 *	0.4 ± 0.1	0.4 ± 0.1	0.011	0.410	0.423
Sit and Stand 30 s (n)	9.2 ± 4.8	6.7 ± 1.7	10.3 ± 2.5	15.2 ± 4.4 *	8.7 ± 2.4	10.0 ± 3.7	0.035	0.470	0.388
Handgrip (Dominant, kg)	20.5 ± 5.7	14.0 ± 7.3	21.4 ± 8.3	20.2 ± 8.0 *	17.3 ± 5.2	17.1 ± 3.8	0.114	0.432	0.827
Handgrip (Non-Dominant, kg)	20.7 ± 5.7	11.7 ± 4.7	20.6 ± 8.4	19.5 ± 7.3	15.6 ± 4.0	15.3 ± 3.4	0.100	0.409	0.838
Muscular									
Frailty Indicator	26.6 ± 8.3	32.4 ± 5.6	23.0 ± 6.3	20.3 ± 6.3	28.8 ± 3.3	27.6 ± 3.7	0.187	0.001	0.106
Concentric Peak Force (kg)	4.8 ± 0.3	4.6 ± 0.6	4.8 ± 0.4	7.0 ± 1.3 *	4.5 ± 0.2	4.9 ± 0.6	0.040	0.043	0.109
Eccentric Peak Force (kg)	3.4 ± 0.2	3.5 ± 0.2	3.4 ± 0.4	4.5 ± 1.1 *	3.3 ± 0.1	3.5 ± 0.1 *	0.046	0.142	0.446

Legend: BMI = Body mass index; CG = Control Group; DCI/BMR = Daily Caloric Intake and Basal Metabolic Rate; EG1 = Experimental group with dynamometer; EG2 = Experimental group with weighted vest; * = sig > 0.05.

The mixed-model ANOVA (2 × 3) showed no significant group × moment interactions for any of the variables related to body composition, physical condition, or muscular capacity (Table 2), indicating that the patterns of change between groups did not differ statistically. However, main effects of group and moment were observed for some variables; therefore, the within-group analyses are presented solely as complementary descriptive information and do not imply differences in the relative effectiveness of the interventions.

3.2. Body Composition

The mixed-model ANOVA revealed no significant group × moment interactions for any body composition variables ($p > 0.05$), indicating that the patterns of change did not differ statistically between groups. Within-group analyses showed that EG1 experienced a small but statistically significant increase in fat-free mass (+2.0 kg, $p < 0.05$) and BMI (+1.2 kg/m^2, $p < 0.05$), while no significant changes were observed in total body fat or body water ($p > 0.05$). Conversely, EG2 exhibited a significant increase in total body fat

https://doi.org/10.3390/healthcare14030303

(+1.2 kg, $p < 0.05$), with no other meaningful changes. The control group (CG) did not present significant variations in any body composition parameter ($p > 0.05$).

3.3. Functional Variables

The mixed-model ANOVA indicated no significant group × moment interactions for physical function (3 m walking speed $p = 0.423$; Sit-to-Stand 30 s $p = 0.388$; handgrip dominant $p = 0.827$; handgrip non-dominant $p = 0.838$). There were main effects of group for walking speed ($p = 0.011$) and Sit-to-Stand ($p = 0.035$), while moment effects were not significant (all $p > 0.40$). Within groups, EG1 improved walking speed (0.5 ± 0.2 to 0.6 ± 0.3 m/s; ≈+0.1 m/s; significant) and Sit-to-Stand performance (10.3 ± 2.5 to 15.2 ± 4.4 repetitions; +4.9; significant). Handgrip (dominant) decreased in EG1 (21.4 ± 8.3 to 20.2 ± 8.0 kg; −1.2 kg; significant), with no significant change in the non-dominant hand (20.6 ± 8.4 to 19.5 ± 7.3 kg). EG2 and CG did not show significant pre–post changes in walking speed or Sit-to-Stand; descriptively, CG walking speed declined (0.5 ± 0.1 to 0.4 ± 0.1 m/s).

3.4. Muscular Capacity

The mixed-model ANOVA revealed no significant group × moment interactions for frailty ($p = 0.106$), concentric peak force ($p = 0.109$), or eccentric peak force ($p = 0.446$). There was a main effect of moment for frailty ($p = 0.001$) and concentric peak force ($p = 0.043$), and main effects of group for concentric ($p = 0.040$) and eccentric peak force ($p = 0.046$). Complementary within-group descriptives showed that EG1 increased concentric peak force (4.8 ± 0.4 to 7.0 ± 1.3 kg; +2.2 kg; significant) and eccentric peak force (3.4 ± 0.4 to 4.5 ± 1.1 kg; +1.1 kg; significant). EG2 increased eccentric peak force (3.3 ± 0.1 to 3.5 ± 0.1 kg; +0.2 kg; significant), with a modest, non-significant rise in concentric force (4.5 ± 0.2 to 4.9 ± 0.6 kg). CG showed a small, non-significant decline in concentric peak force (4.8 ± 0.3 to 4.6 ± 0.6 kg) and a slight increase in eccentric force (3.4 ± 0.2 to 3.5 ± 0.2 kg). Frailty scores worsened descriptively in CG (26.6 ± 8.3 to 32.4 ± 5.6) and improved in EG1 (23.0 ± 6.3 to 20.3 ± 6.3) and EG2 (28.8 ± 3.3 to 27.6 ± 3.7), consistent with the moment main effect but not supported by a significant interaction.

Post hoc Bonferroni comparisons (Table 3) revealed no statistically significant differences between EG1 and CG in walking speed ($p = 0.053$), although EG2 performed significantly better than EG1 (mean difference = −0.31 m/s, $p = 0.005$). The comparison between EG2 and CG was not significant ($p = 1.000$). For the Sit-to-Stand test, EG1 performed significantly better than CG (mean difference = 7.13 repetitions, $p = 0.017$), whereas the difference between EG1 and EG2 did not reach statistical significance ($p = 0.076$). Regarding frailty, EG1 showed significantly lower frailty scores compared with CG (mean difference = −13.25, $p < 0.001$), and EG2 also performed significantly better than CG (mean difference = −8.83, $p = 0.008$), with no significant difference between EG1 and EG2 ($p = 0.125$). For neuromuscular outcomes, EG1 demonstrated significantly greater concentric peak force than both CG (mean difference = 1.60 kg, $p = 0.030$) and EG2 (mean difference = 1.40 kg, p = 0.016). In terms of eccentric peak force, EG2 showed significantly higher values than EG1 (mean difference = −0.95 kg, $p = 0.026$), whereas the difference between EG1 and CG did not reach statistical significance ($p = 0.157$).

https://doi.org/10.3390/healthcare14030303

Table 3. Post-Anova Intervention-up Test Using Bonferroni.

Multiple Comparison								
Dependent Variable		Groups	Groups	Mean Difference	Std Error	Sig.	95% Confidence Interval Lower Limit	Upper Limit
3 m Walking speed (m/s)	Bonferroni	EG1	CG	0.2714	0.10190	0.053	−0.0031	0.5458
			EG2	0.3089	0.08086	0.005	0.0911	0.5267
		CG	EG1	−0.2714	0.10190	0.053	−0.5458	0.0031
			EG2	0.0375	0.09999	1.000	−0.2318	0.3069
		EG2	EG1	−0.3089	0.08086	0.005	−0.5267	−0.0911
			CG	−0.0375	0.09999	1.000	−0.3069	0.2318
Sit and Stand 30 s (n)	Bonferroni	EG1	CG	7.1250	2.20605	0.017	1.1825	13.0675
			EG2	4.3472	1.75048	0.076	−0.3681	9.0626
		CG	EG1	−7.1250	2.20605	0.017	−13.0675	−1.1825
			EG2	−2.7778	2.16481	0.657	−8.6092	3.0537
		EG2	EG1	−4.3472	1.75048	0.076	−9.0626	0.3681
			CG	2.7778	2.16481	0.657	−3.0537	8.6092
			CG	0.7778	3.81323	1.000	−9.4941	11.0496
Frailty Indicator	Bonferroni	EG1	CG	−13.2500	2.49727	<0.001	−19.9770	−6.5230
			EG2	−4.4167	1.98156	0.125	−9.7545	0.9211
		CG	EG1	13.2500	2.49727	<0.001	6.5230	19.9770
			EG2	8.8333	2.45059	0.008	2.2321	15.4346
		EG2	EG1	4.4167	1.98156	0.125	−0.9211	9.7545
			CG	−8.8333	2.45059	0.008	−15.4346	−2.2321
Concentric Peak Force (kg)	Bonferroni	EG1	CG	1.5963 *	0.54189	0.030	0.1365	3.0560
			EG2	1.3999 *	0.42998	0.016	0.2416	2.5581
		CG	EG1	−1.5963 *	0.54189	0.030	−3.0560	−0.1365
			EG2	−0.1964	0.53176	1.000	−1.6288	1.2360
		EG2	EG1	−1.3999 *	0.42998	0.016	−2.5581	−0.2416
			CG	0.1964	0.53176	1.000	−1.2360	1.6288
Eccentric Peak Force (kg)	Bonferroni	EG1	CG	0.8313	0.39435	0.157	−0.2310	1.8935
			EG2	0.9460 *	0.31291	0.026	0.1031	1.7889
		CG	EG1	−0.8313	0.39435	0.157	−1.8935	0.2310
			EG2	0.1147	0.38698	1.000	−0.9277	1.1571
		EG2	EG1	−0.9460 *	0.31291	0.026	−1.7889	−0.1031
			CG	−0.1147	0.38698	1.000	−1.1571	0.9277

Legend: CG = Control Group; EG1 = Experimental group with dynamometer; EG2 = Experimental group with weighted vest; * = sig < 0.05.

3.5. Relationship Between Walking Speed and Peak Eccentric Force

Figure 2 illustrates the effects of the intervention on peak eccentric force and its relationship with walking speed in the strength training groups. In the post-test, EG1 demonstrated better application of eccentric force; higher walking speed corresponded to greater eccentric force application, while EG2 did not display stable behavior. EG1 utilized higher values of eccentric force during walking. Both experimental groups increased peak eccentric force. In the post-test, EG1 exhibited a stronger association between eccentric peak force and walking speed, suggesting a potential relationship between neuromuscular adaptations and functional performance; however, causal inferences cannot be established.

4. Discussion

The objective of this pilot study was to analyze the effects of two strength interventions focusing on the eccentric phase on peak strength (concentric and eccentric) in older adults residing in a nursing home, as well as to assess their impact on functional capacity and health-related indicators of frailty and independence.

The main findings highlight that EG1 achieved significant improvements in concentric and eccentric peak force, walking speed, and chair stand performance, while EG2 showed smaller gains. The mixed-model ANOVA did not reveal significant group × moment interactions for concentric or eccentric peak force. However, significant main effects of group and Bonferroni-adjusted post hoc comparisons supported between-group differences in concentric peak force. Therefore, differential intervention effects between groups cannot be statistically established. Although significant main effects of group and Bonferroni-adjusted post hoc comparisons were observed for concentric peak force, these findings should be interpreted with caution and do not indicate superiority of one intervention

https://doi.org/10.3390/healthcare14030303

over another. These results are consistent with previous studies emphasizing the role of eccentric training in enhancing neuromuscular efficiency [20] and functional independence in older adults [24,25], particularly at the within-group level.

Frailty indicators decreased in EG1, although not reaching statistical significance, while Bonferroni comparisons confirmed that EG1 differed significantly from CG. This supports the idea that even modest changes in frailty scores may translate into meaningful health gains, as reported by Studenski et al. [2] and van Kan et al. [6], who identified gait speed and frailty indicators as predictors of hospitalization, falls, and loss of autonomy. Our results suggest that short-term, low-frequency resistance training using a functional electromechanical dynamometer (FEMD) may represent a promising strategy for addressing frailty-related outcomes, supporting independence, and improving quality of life, in line with previous evidence on functional resistance training [3,4]. However, these results derive from a very small sample size and therefore are not generalizable to broader populations.

The improvements in walking speed observed in this study, together with gains in eccentric and concentric force, underscore the potential of tailored strength training as a non-pharmacological intervention for maintaining health, independence, and well-being among frail older adults.

This agrees with findings from Cadore et al. [4] and Fragala et al. [51], emphasized that muscle power and walking speed are critical markers of functional capacity and predictors of adverse outcomes. In our study, Bonferroni tests confirmed significant differences between EG1 and EG2 in walking speed, suggesting a potential functional advantage of FEMD-based training for mobility-related outcomes.

These findings reinforce that functional resistance training may represent a low-cost and sustainable approach, as highlighted by Tou et al. [52] and Ramírez-Campillo et al. [53], demonstrated that high-speed resistance training improves functionality in frail and pre-frail older adults.

All participants performed the same eight exercises twice a week for 8 weeks. The only methodological difference between the two groups was the use of a weighted vest or a cord during the sit-to-stand exercise. The results indicate that both interventions achieved statistically significant differences in peak eccentric strength, with EG1 also showing improvements in concentric strength. This supports the idea that eccentric-focused interventions are particularly effective, consistent with Caserotti et al. [23] and Roig et al. [24].

The second objective was to determine whether strength improvements affected functional capacity in sedentary and older adults residing in a nursing home; in this case, the intervention with the FEMD resulted in significant improvements in the Chair Stand Test. These findings suggest that the intervention applied in EG1 was associated with improvements in selected functional outcomes, as strength gains were accompanied by improvements in walking speed and performance in the sit-to-stand task [46,54]—both of which are key indicators of mobility and independence in older adults.

In terms of body composition, no significant differences were observed between pre- and post-intervention measurements in the control group. In contrast, EG1 demonstrated increases in both body weight and BMI without a corresponding increase in fat mass, suggesting that these changes may be attributable to gains in fat-free mass. Although an increase in fat-free mass was observed in EG1, it did not reach statistical significance, possibly due to the small sample size or the short duration of the intervention.

Despite the potential impact on public health, there are few interventions aimed at mitigating the decline in functional capacity among institutionalized populations [38]. Physical activity, particularly strength training, is a crucial strategy for preventing or

https://doi.org/10.3390/healthcare14030303

delaying frailty in older adults. Current literature highlights that high-speed resistance training is effective for improving functionality in older adults [4,5,52,53], as muscle power is a more sensitive predictor of functional capacity than isolated maximum strength. The results of this study support this exercise prescription, as EG1 demonstrated improvements in both peak concentric and eccentric force, while EG2 showed smaller improvements.

To our knowledge, this is the first intervention conducted with a FEMD in older adults residing in a nursing home. The use of this device appears to offer advantages in controlling load throughout the movement (particularly during the eccentric phase), which may explain the greater within-group gains in peak strength were observed in EG1 (46.5% concentric; 34% eccentric) compared with EG2, although these differences should be interpreted cautiously due to the absence of significant group × moment interactions (4.4% and 6.1%, respectively). The differences between the two interventions likely lie in biomechanical aspects and execution, as using the FEMD requires participants to remain under tension longer, especially in the eccentric phase, potentially enhancing body awareness and control throughout the movement. This may facilitate optimal progressive overload and an increasing workload, generating greater mechanical tension through Maximum Voluntary Contraction (MVC).

The improvement in strength gains induced by training is also associated with enhancements in muscular function. EG1 showed significant improvements in the 30 s sit-to-stand test and walking speed, while EG2 did not exhibit significant differences in these tests. In this context, several studies [54–56] advocate for the use of rapid execution training to maximize the effects of exercise therapies in older individuals, including the oldest old [57]. Reid & Fielding [58] explain that power—the ability to generate force quickly—is crucial for performing daily movements and responding to situations requiring rapid reactions, such as preventing falls. They highlight how this type of training can induce neural changes in muscle recruitment that transfer to both isometric and dynamic exercises [56,59]. Lavin et al. [60] suggest that neuromuscular aging can be inhibited by improving motor unit integrity, and corticospinal excitability, while Maki & McIlroy [61] emphasized the importance of rapid torque generation for balance recovery.

Regarding training with a weighted vest, the study by Mierzwick [62] reported improvements in certain strength variables but no significant differences in the five-time sit-to-stand test. One explanation is that the load from the vest applies to the trunk and pelvis rather than directly to the lower limb. Pagan et al. [35] also noted that vest training provides overload benefits when worn during daily activities or aerobic resistance, but not for maximum strength improvement.

In terms of upper body strength, no improvements were observed in either EG1 or EG2, as seen in other studies [63,64]. Furthermore, the EG1 group exhibited a decrease in hand grip strength in the dominant hand. This decrease could be attributed to the greater emphasis on overload for other body parts, with insufficient direct stimulation of the forearm and hand musculature due to the use of bands and the sets and repetitions outlined in this study. This highlights the importance of including specific exercises for upper limb strength if improvement in this area is desired, as Valdés-Badilla et al. [63] and Chen et al. [64] also reported limited gains in grip strength when upper limb training was not specifically targeted.

Concerning frailty, there was a trend toward improvement in EG1 (decreasing from 23.00 to 20.33, $t = 2.090$, $p = 0.091$), although it did not reach statistical significance. This suggests that longer interventions or larger samples may be required to achieve statistical significance. Nevertheless, even small individual improvements in frailty scores can represent meaningful gains in daily life, as gait speed and frailty indices are strongly associated with autonomy and hospitalization risk [2,6].

https://doi.org/10.3390/healthcare14030303

The control group showed no significant changes in any evaluated parameters, including body composition, physical condition, and muscular capacity. This supports the idea that strength training is the determining factor for the improvements observed in EG1, as the absence of training stimulus resulted in no modifications in the evaluated variables. Moreover, the strength gains in EG2 did not reach a minimal effective load necessary to translate into improvements in functional capacities that influence the quality of life of older adults.

Walking speed has been recognized in scientific literature as a key marker of functional capacity and overall health, particularly in older adult populations. Studies have reported that increases in muscle power contribute to improved force generation speed, associated with greater walking speed, better quality of life, and reduced frailty (or lower risk of hospitalization, falls, and loss of autonomy) [2,6,51].

In our study, the correlation between eccentric peak force and walking speed was confirmed, reinforcing the idea [26,51] that eccentric adaptations are critical for mobility improvements.

The current results, demonstrating that even with a frequency of two sessions per week, significant improvements in muscle strength can be achieved, which is essential for maintaining autonomy in this population. During the eccentric phase, the muscle lengthens while maintaining activated actin and myosin bridges under tension. This process not only controls impact upon ground contact but also stores elastic energy in muscle and tendon structures. This energy is then released in the concentric phase, where the muscle shortens to propel movement. This interaction is key to movement efficiency and economy. The improved application of force during movement appears to stem from enhanced Stretch-Shortening Cycle capabilities in those who trained with the dynamometer compared to those who underwent weighted vest training. One possible explanation for these gains may be that participants using the dynamometer experienced more time under tension than those training with the vest [17]. Therefore, gains in the eccentric phase, along with those in the concentric phase, may have led to improvements in functional tests (greater capacity to transfer forces) [26]. Inability to fully activate a muscle occurs when there is inadequate neural input for a muscle or when excitation-contraction coupling is insufficient to ensure that all muscle motor units are active and firing at the appropriate maximum frequency [59]. Conversely, the EG2 group demonstrated less stable behavior, indicating that adaptations in the stretch-shortening cycle (and thus in eccentric phase effectiveness) were neither consistent nor significant. In conclusion, it can be suggested that improvements in eccentric strength optimize the transition to the concentric phase, allowing for more effective utilization of stored elastic energy. However, improvements in the concentric phase are also necessary for enhancing functional capacity in dependent and institutionalized older adults.

This study has several limitations that should be considered when interpreting the results. First, the small sample size and the presence of various comorbidities—particularly those related to cognitive impairment—limited the ability to maintain strict control over training load and adherence. Additionally, the absence of dietary monitoring or nutritional intervention may have influenced the outcomes related to body composition. Finally, the lack of post-intervention follow-up makes it difficult to assess the long-term sustainability of the improvements achieved.

Another possible limitation is the "attention effect" in the control group, since participants may benefit from social interaction or minimal activity even without structured training. Future studies should consider allowing control groups to engage in light activities (e.g., social gatherings, stretching) to minimize this bias. Moreover, the absence

https://doi.org/10.3390/healthcare14030303

of blinding for evaluators represents another methodological limitation that should be addressed in subsequent trials.

5. Conclusions

This pilot study suggests that eccentric-focused strength training performed with a functional electromechanical dynamometer is associated with neuromuscular improvements, particularly in concentric peak force, in frail nursing home residents. However, no significant group × moment interactions were observed, indicating that differential training effects between interventions cannot be established. Post hoc between-group comparisons therefore reflect cross-sectional differences rather than training-induced superiority. Functional improvements should be interpreted cautiously.

FEMD-based training may represent a promising functional strength training strategy for institutionalized older adults. Future randomized controlled trials with larger samples and longer follow-up are required to confirm these findings.

Author Contributions: Conceptualization, H.V.; methodology, H.V. and J.M.C.; formal analysis, J.M.C.; Data curation and writing—original draft preparation H.V. and J.M.C.; Writing—review and editing, H.V., C.F., Á.R.-P., V.S.-G. and Ó.G.-G. visualization and supervision, H.V., C.F., L.J.C., V.S.-G., Ó.G.-G., D.J.-M., Á.R.-P. and J.M.C. All authors have read and agreed to the published version of the manuscript.

Funding: This study was funded by the Consejo Superior de Deportes (Project code: CSD2025_104947), Universidad de Granada, and the Red de Dinamometría Funcional Deportiva.

Institutional Review Board Statement: The study design and protocol adhered to the tenets of the Declaration of Helsinki and was approved by the University Review Board (CEIC-14-1009-17), approval date 26 September 2017.

Informed Consent Statement: Informed consent was obtained from all subjects involved in the study.

Data Availability Statement: The data supporting the findings of this study are not publicly available due to ethical and privacy restrictions related to the protection of participants' personal data. The data may be made available from the corresponding author upon reasonable request and with approval from the relevant ethics committee.

Acknowledgments: The authors are grateful to all the older adults who participated in this study. We would also like to extend our sincere thanks to the director and physiotherapist of the DOMUSVI nursing home in the city of Pontevedra for their collaboration and support. Finally, we thank the students of the Bachelor's Degree in Physical Activity and Sports Sciences for their valuable assistance.

Conflicts of Interest: The authors declare no conflicts of interest.

References

1. Hoogendijk, E.O.; Afilalo, J.; Ensrud, K.E.; Kowal, P.; Onder, G.; Fried, L.P. Frailty: Implications for clinical practice and public health. *Lancet* **2019**, *394*, 1365–1375. [CrossRef]
2. Studenski, S.; Perera, S.; Patel, K.; Rosano, C.; Faulkner, K.; Inzitari, M.; Brach, J.; Chandler, J.; Cawthon, P.; Connor, B.E.; et al. Gait Speed and Survival in Older Adults. *Jama-J. Am. Med. Assoc.* **2011**, *305*, 50–58. [CrossRef]
3. Navarrete-Villanueva, D.; Gomez-Cabello, A.; Marin-Puyalto, J.; Moreno, L.A.; Vicente-Rodriguez, G.; Casajus, J.A. Frailty and Physical Fitness in Elderly People: A Systematic Review and Meta-analysis. *Sports Med.* **2021**, *51*, 143–160. [CrossRef]
4. Cadore, E.L.; Rodriguez-Manas, L.; Sinclair, A.; Izquierdo, M. Effects of different exercise interventions on risk of falls, gait ability, and balance in physically frail older adults: A systematic review. *Rejuvenation Res.* **2013**, *16*, 105–114. [CrossRef]
5. Cadore, E.L.; Izquierdo, M. Muscle Power Training: A Hallmark for Muscle Function Retaining in Frail Clinical Setting. *J. Am. Med. Dir. Assoc.* **2018**, *19*, 190–192. [CrossRef]

https://doi.org/10.3390/healthcare14030303

6. Van Kan, G.A.; Rolland, Y.; Andrieu, S.; Bauer, J.; Beauchet, O.; Bonnefoy, M.; Cesari, M.; Donini, L.; Gillette-Guyonnet, S.; Inzitari, M.; et al. Gait Speed at Usual Pace as a Predictor of Adverse Outcomes in Community-Dwelling Older People an International Academy on Nutrition and Aging (Iana) Task Force. *J. Nutr. Health Aging* **2009**, *13*, 881–889. [CrossRef]
7. Bean, J.; Herman, S.; Kiely, D.K.; Callahan, D.; Mizer, K.; Frontera, W.R.; Fielding, R.A. Weighted stair climbing in mobility-limited older people: A pilot study. *J. Am. Geriatr. Soc.* **2002**, *50*, 663–670. [CrossRef]
8. Bull, F.C.; Al-Ansari, S.S.; Biddle, S.; Borodulin, K.; Buman, M.P.; Cardon, G.; Carty, C.; Chaput, J.-P.; Chastin, S.; Chou, R.; et al. World Health Organization 2020 guidelines on physical activity and sedentary behaviour. *Br. J. Sports Med.* **2020**, *54*, 1451–1462. [CrossRef] [PubMed]
9. Petnehazy, N.; Barnes, H.N.; Newman, A.B.; Kritchevsky, S.B.; Cummings, S.R.; Hepple, R.T.; Cawthon, P.M. Muscle Mass, Strength, Power and Physical Performance and Their Association with Quality of Life in Older Adults, the Study of Muscle, Mobility and Aging (SOMMA). *J. Frality Aging* **2024**, *13*, 384–390. [CrossRef] [PubMed]
10. Bean, J.F.; Kiely, D.K.; Herman, S.; Leveille, S.G.; Mizer, K.; Frontera, W.R.; Fielding, R.A. The relationship between leg power and physical performance in mobility-limited older people. *J. Am. Geriatr. Soc.* **2002**, *50*, 461–467.
11. Garber, C.E.; Blissmer, B.; Deschenes, M.R.; Deschenes, M.R.; Franklin, B.A.; Lamonte, M.J.; Lee, I.-M.; Nieman, D.C.; Swain, D.P. Quantity and Quality of Exercise for Developing and Maintaining Cardiorespiratory, Musculoskeletal, and Neuromotor Fitness in Apparently Healthy Adults: Guidance for Prescribing Exercise. *Med. Sci. Sports Exerc.* **2011**, *43*, 1334–1359. [CrossRef]
12. Van Roie, E.; Walker, S.; Van Driessche, S.; Delabastita, T.; Vanwanseele, B.; Delecluse, C. An age-adapted plyometric exercise program improves dynamic strength, jump performance and functional capacity in older men either similarly or more than traditional resistance training. *PLoS ONE* **2020**, *15*, e0237921. [CrossRef]
13. Shumway-Cook, A.; Silver, I.F.; LeMier, M.; York, S.; Cummings, P.; Koepsell, T.D. Effectiveness of a community-based multifactorial intervention on falls and fall risk factors in community-living older adults: A randomized, controlled trial. *J. Gerontol. Ser. A* **2007**, *62*, 1420–1427. [CrossRef]
14. Fiatarone, M.A.; Marks, E.C.; Ryan, N.D.; Meredith, C.N.; Lipsitz, L.A.; Evans, W.J. High-Intensity Strength Training in Nonagenarians—Effects on Skeletal-Muscle. *Jama-J. Am. Med. Assoc.* **1990**, *263*, 3029–3034. [CrossRef]
15. Latham, N.K.; Anderson, C.S.; Lee, A.; Bennett, D.A.; Moseley, A.; Cameron, I.D. For the Fitness Collaborative Group. A randomized, controlled trial of quadriceps resistance exercise and vitamin D in frail older people: The Frailty Interventions Trial in Elderly Subjects (FITNESS). *J. Am. Geriatr. Soc.* **2003**, *51*, 291–299. [CrossRef] [PubMed]
16. García-Pinillos, F.; Martínez-Amat, A.; Hita-Contreras, F.; Martínez-López, E.J.; Latorre-Román, P.A. Effects of a Contrast Training Program without External Load on Vertical Jump, Kicking Speed, Sprint, and Agility of Young Soccer Players. *J. Strength Cond. Res.* **2014**, *28*, 2452–2460. [CrossRef] [PubMed]
17. Jimenez-Lupion, D.; Chirosa-Rios, I.; Lizama-Perez, R.; Chirosa-Rios, L.; Jerez-Mayorga, D. A Novel Method for Assessing Load-Velocity Profiles with a Motorized Resistance Device in the Sit-to-Stand Test in Older Adults. *J. Strength Cond. Res.* **2025**, *39*, e1112–e1118. [CrossRef]
18. Rodríguez-Perea, A.; Jerez-Mayorga, D.; García-Ramos, A.; Martínez-García, D.; Ríos, L.J.C. Reliability and concurrent validity of a functional electromechanical dynamometer device for the assessment of movement velocity. *Proc. Inst. Mech. Eng. Part P J. Sports Eng. Technol.* **2021**, *235*, 176–181. [CrossRef]
19. Schoenfeld, B.J.; Ogborn, D.I.; Vigotsky, A.D.; Franchi, M.V.; Krieger, J.W. Hypertrophic Effects of Concentric vs. Eccentric Muscle Actions: A Systematic Review and Meta-Analysis. *J. Strength Cond. Res.* **2017**, *31*, 2599–2608. [CrossRef] [PubMed]
20. Douglas, J.; Pearson, S.; Ross, A.; McGuigan, M. Effects of Accentuated Eccentric Loading on Muscle Properties, Strength, Power, and Speed in Resistance-Trained Rugby Players. *J. Strength Cond. Res.* **2018**, *32*, 2750–2761. [CrossRef]
21. Diong, J.; Carden, P.C.; O'Sullivan, K.; Sherrington, C.; Reed, D.S. Eccentric exercise improves joint flexibility in adults: A systematic review update and meta-analysis. *Musculoskelet. Sci. Pract.* **2022**, *60*, 102556. [CrossRef]
22. Menz, H.B.; Auhl, M.; Spink, M.J. Foot problems as a risk factor for falls in community-dwelling older people: A systematic review and meta-analysis. *Maturitas* **2018**, *118*, 7–14. [CrossRef]
23. Caserotti, P.; Aagaard, P.; Puggaard, L. Changes in power and force generation during coupled eccentric-concentric versus concentric muscle contraction with training and aging. *Eur. J. Appl. Physiol.* **2008**, *103*, 151–161. [CrossRef]
24. Roig, M.; O'bRien, K.; Kirk, G.; Murray, R.; McKinnon, P.; Shadgan, B.; Reid, W.D. The effects of eccentric versus concentric resistance training on muscle strength and mass in healthy adults: A systematic review with meta-analysis. *Br. J. Sports Med.* **2009**, *43*, 556–568. [CrossRef] [PubMed]
25. Lepley, L.K.; Lepley, A.S.; Onate, J.A.; Grooms, D.R. Eccentric Exercise to Enhance Neuromuscular Control. *Sports Health* **2017**, *9*, 333–340. [CrossRef]
26. Naczk, M.; Marszalek, S.; Naczk, A. Inertial Training Improves Strength, Balance, and Gait Speed in Elderly Nursing Home Residents. *Clin. Interv. Aging* **2020**, *15*, 177–184. [CrossRef]
27. Baxter, B.A.; Baross, A.W.; Ryan, D.J.; Wright, B.H.; Kay, A.D. The acute and repeated bout effects of multi-joint eccentric exercise on physical function and balance in older adults. *Eur. J. Appl. Physiol.* **2023**, *123*, 2131–2143. [CrossRef]

 https://doi.org/10.3390/healthcare14030303

28. Torgerson, D.J.; Sibbald, B. Understanding controlled trials. What is a patient preference trial? *Br. Med. J.* **1998**, *316*, 360. [CrossRef] [PubMed]
29. Lauzâ, M.; Martel, D.D.; Agnoux, A.; Sirois, M.J.; Daoust, R. Feasibility, acceptability and effects of a home-based exercise program using a gerontechnology on physical capacities after a minor injury in community-living older adults: A pilot study. *J. Nutr. Health Aging* **2018**, *22*, 16–25. [CrossRef] [PubMed]
30. Palencia, N.M.A.; Martínez, M.S.; Herráiz, M.M.G.; Arribas, S.A.; García, A.G.; Bueno, C.A. La actividad física vigorosa se relaciona con menor adiposidad y una condición física saludables en niños de 9–10 años. *Rev. Andal. Med. Deporte* **2015**, *8*, 38. [CrossRef]
31. Del-Cuerpo, I.; Jerez-Mayorga, D.; Delgado-Floody, P.; Morenas-Aguilar, M.D.; Chirosa-Ríos, L.J. Test-Retest Reliability of the Functional Electromechanical Dynamometer for Squat Exercise. *Int. J. Environ. Res. Public Health* **2023**, *20*, 1289. [CrossRef]
32. Reyes-Ferrada, W.; Chirosa-Ríos, L.; Chirosa-Ríos, I.; Martínez-García, D.; Barboza-Gonzalez, P.; Ulloa-Díaz, D.; Jerez-Mayorga, D.; Rodríguez-Perea, Á. A new reliable device to assess trunk extensors strength. *Acta Bioeng. Biomech.* **2022**, *24*, 39–47. [CrossRef]
33. DeFreitas, J.M.; Beck, T.W.; Stock, M.S.; Dillon, M.A.; Kasishke, P.R. An examination of the time course of training-induced skeletal muscle hypertrophy. *Eur. J. Appl. Physiol.* **2011**, *111*, 2785–2790. [CrossRef]
34. Stock, M.S.; Mota, J.A.; DeFranco, R.N.; Grue, K.A.; Jacobo, A.U.; Chung, E.; Moon, J.R.; DeFreitas, J.M.; Beck, T.W. The time course of short-term hypertrophy in the absence of eccentric muscle damage. *Eur. J. Appl. Physiol.* **2017**, *117*, 989–1004. [CrossRef] [PubMed]
35. Pagan, J.I.; Bradshaw, B.A.; Bejte, B.; Hart, J.N.; Perez, V.; Knowles, K.S.; Beausejour, J.P.; Luzadder, M.; Menger, R.; Osorio, C.; et al. Task-specific resistance training adaptations in older adults: Comparing traditional and functional exercise interventions. *Front. Aging-Lausanne* **2024**, *5*, 1335534. [CrossRef]
36. Bevan, A.; Vidoni, E.; Watts, A. Rate of Perceived Exertion and Cardiorespiratory Fitness in Older Adults with and without Alzheimer's Disease. *Int. J. Exerc. Sci.* **2020**, *13*, 18–35. [CrossRef]
37. García-García, F.J.; Carnicero, J.A.; Losa-Reyna, J.; Alfaro-Acha, A.; Castillo-Gallego, C.; Rosado-Artalejo, C.; Gutiérrrez-Ávila, G.; Rodriguez-Mañas, L. Frailty Trait Scale-Short Form: A Frailty Instrument for Clinical Practice. *J. Am. Med. Dir. Assoc.* **2020**, *21*, 1260–1266.e2. [CrossRef]
38. Raymond, M.J.; Jeffs, K.J.; Winter, A.; Soh, S.E.; Hunter, P.; Holland, A.E. The effects of a high-intensity functional exercise group on clinical outcomes in hospitalised older adults: An assessor-blinded, randomised-controlled trial. *Age Ageing* **2017**, *46*, 208–213. [CrossRef]
39. Brach, J.S.; Perera, S.; Shuman, V.; Gil, A.B.; Kriska, A.; Nadkarni, N.K.; Rockette-Wagner, B.; Cham, R.; VanSwearingen, J.M. Effect of Timing and Coordination Training on Mobility and Physical Activity Among Community-Dwelling Older Adults: A Randomized Clinical Trial. *JAMA Netw. Open* **2022**, *5*, e2212921. [CrossRef] [PubMed]
40. Stewart, A.; Marfell-Jones, M.; Olds, T.; Ridden, H. *International Standards for Anthropometric Assessment*, 3rd ed.; Lower-Hunt: Nordinsel, New Zealand, 2011.
41. Verney, J.; Schwartz, C.; Amiche, S.; Pereira, B.; Thivel, D. Comparisons of a Multi-Frequency Bioelectrical Impedance Analysis to the Dual-Energy X-Ray Absorptiometry Scan in Healthy Young Adults Depending on their Physical Activity Level. *J. Hum. Kinet.* **2015**, *47*, 73–80. [CrossRef]
42. Ayeser, T.; Basak, M.; Arslan, K.; Sayan, I. Investigating the correlation of the number of diagnostic criteria to serum adiponectin, leptin, resistin, TNF-alpha, EGFR levels and abdominal adipose tissue. *Diabetes Metab. Synd.* **2016**, *10*, S165–S169. [CrossRef]
43. Garatachez, N.; de Paz-Fernández, J.A. Cuantificación de la actividad física en personas mayores. *Rev. Española Geriatr. Gerontol.* **2005**, *40*, 47–52. [CrossRef]
44. Allen, D.; Barnett, F. Reliability and validity of an electronic dynamometer for measuring grip strength. *Int. J. Ther. Rehabil.* **2011**, *18*, 258–264. [CrossRef]
45. Lee, S.C.; Wu, L.C.; Chiang, S.L.; Lu, L.H.; Chen, C.Y.; Lin, C.H.; Ni, C.H.; Lin, C.H. Validating the Capability for Measuring Age-Related Changes in Grip-Force Strength Using a Digital Hand-Held Dynamometer in Healthy Young and Elderly Adults. *Biomed Res. Int.* **2020**, *2020*, 6936879. [CrossRef]
46. Jones, C.J.; Rikli, R.E.; Beam, W.C.A. 30-s chair-stand test as a measure of lower body strength in community-residing older adults. *Res. Q. Exerc. Sport* **1999**, *70*, 113–119. [CrossRef] [PubMed]
47. Lyons, J.G.; Heeren, T.; Stuver, S.O.; Fredman, L. Assessing the Agreement Between 3-Meter and 6-Meter Walk Tests in 136 Community-Dwelling Older Adults. *J. Aging Health* **2015**, *27*, 594–605. [CrossRef] [PubMed]
48. Jimenez-Lupion, D.; Chirosa-Rios, I.; Lizama-Perez, R.; Chirosa-Rios, L.; Jerez-Mayorga, D. Assessment of muscle function deterioration in aging populations: Insights from the load-velocity relationship during the loaded sit-to-stand test. *Exp. Gerontol.* **2025**, *206*, 112767. [CrossRef]
49. Sousa, N.; Mendes, R.; Abrantes, C.; Sampaio, J.; Oliveira, J. Effectiveness of combined exercise training to improve functional fitness in older adults: A randomized controlled trial. *Geriatr. Gerontol. Int.* **2014**, *14*, 892–898. [CrossRef]
50. Chan, Y. Biostatistics 301A. Repeated measurement analysis. *Singap. Med. J.* **2004**, *45*, 457.

 https://doi.org/10.3390/healthcare14030303

51. Fragala, M.S.; Cadore, E.L.; Dorgo, S.; Izquierdo, M.; Kraemer, W.J.; Peterson, M.D.; Ryan, E.D. Resistance Training for Older Adults: Position Statement from the National Strength and Conditioning Association. *J. Strength Cond. Res.* **2019**, *33*, 2019–2052. [CrossRef]
52. Tou, N.X.; Wee, S.L.; Seah, W.T.; Ng, D.H.M.; Pang, B.W.J.; Lau, L.K.; Ng, T.P. Effectiveness of Community-Delivered Functional Power Training Program for Frail and Pre-frail Community-Dwelling Older Adults: A Randomized Controlled Study. *Prev. Sci.* **2021**, *22*, 1048–1059. [CrossRef]
53. Ramírez-Campillo, R.; Castillo, A.; de la Fuente, C.I.; Campos-Jara, C.; Andrade, D.C.; Alvarez, C.; Martínez, C.; Castro-Sepúlveda, M.; Pereira, A.; Marques, M.C.; et al. High-speed resistance training is more effective than low-speed resistance training to increase functional capacity and muscle performance in older women. *Exp. Gerontol.* **2014**, *58*, 51–57. [CrossRef]
54. Pereira, A.; Izquierdo, M.; Silva, A.J.; Costa, A.M.; Bastos, E.; Gonzalez-Badillo, J.J.; Marques, M.C. Effects of high-speed power training on functional capacity and muscle performance in older women. *Exp. Gerontol.* **2012**, *47*, 250–255. [CrossRef] [PubMed]
55. Caserotti, P.; Aagaard, P.; Buttrup Larsen, J.; Puggaard, L. Explosive heavy-resistance training in old and very old adults: Changes in rapid muscle force, strength and power. *Scand. J. Med. Sci. Spor.* **2008**, *18*, 773–782. [CrossRef]
56. Lopes, P.B.; Pereira, G.; Lodovico, A.; Bento, P.C.B.; Rodacki, A.L.F. Strength and Power Training Effects on Lower Limb Force, Functional Capacity, and Static and Dynamic Balance in Older Female Adults. *Rejuvenation Res.* **2016**, *19*, 385–393. [CrossRef]
57. Basco, M.D. Use of a High-Intensity Resistance Exercise Program to Improve Lower Extremity Strength and Mobility in a 105-Year Older Woman: A Case Report. *J. Frality Aging* **2020**, *9*, 122–123. [CrossRef] [PubMed]
58. Reid, K.F.; Fielding, R.A. Skeletal Muscle Power: A Critical Determinant of Physical Functioning in Older Adults. *Exerc. Sport Sci. Rev.* **2012**, *40*, 4–12. [CrossRef] [PubMed]
59. Barry, B.K.; Carson, R.G. The consequences of resistance training for movement control in older adults. *J. Gerontol. Ser. A Biol. Sci. Med. Sci.* **2004**, *59*, 730–754. [CrossRef]
60. Lavin, K.M.; Roberts, B.M.; Fry, C.S.; Moro, T.; Rasmussen, B.B.; Bamman, M.M. The Importance of Resistance Exercise Training to Combat Neuromuscular Aging. *Physiology* **2019**, *34*, 112–122. [CrossRef]
61. Maki, B.E.; McIlroy, W.E. Control of rapid limb movements for balance recovery: Age-related changes and implications for fall prevention. *Age Ageing* **2006**, *35*, ii12–ii18. [CrossRef]
62. Mierzwicki, J.T. Weighted Vest Training in Community-Dwelling Older Adults: A Randomized, Controlled Pilot Study. *Phys. Act. Health* **2019**, *3*, 108–116. [CrossRef]
63. Valdés-Badilla, P.; Guzmán-Muñoz, E.; Hernandez-Martinez, J.; Núñez-Espinosa, C.; Delgado-Floody, P.; Herrera-Valenzuela, T.; Branco, B.H.M.; Zapata-Bastias, J.; Nobari, H. Effectiveness of elastic band training and group-based dance on physical-functional performance in older women with sarcopenia: A pilot study. *BMC Public Health* **2023**, *23*, 2113. [CrossRef]
64. Chen, R.J.; Wu, Q.W.; Wang, D.Y.; Li, Z.; Liu, H.W.; Liu, G.T.; Cui, Y.; Song, L.L. Effects of elastic band exercise on the frailty states in pre-frail elderly people. *Physiother. Theory Pract.* **2020**, *36*, 1000–1008. [CrossRef] [PubMed]

 https://doi.org/10.3390/healthcare14030303

healthcare

MDPI

Article

Acute Effects of a Mini-Trampoline Training Session for Improving Normalized Symmetry Index in Participants with Higher Baseline Inter-Limb Asymmetry

Olga Papale [1,2], Emanuel Festino [1,2], Marianna De Maio [1,2], Francesca Di Rocco [1,2,3], Silvia Zema [1,2], Cristina Cortis [1,2,*] and Andrea Fusco [4]

1 Department of Human Sciences, Society and Health, University of Cassino and Lazio Meridionale, 03043 Cassino, Italy; olga.papale@unicas.it (O.P.); emanuel.festino@unicas.it (E.F.); marianna.demaio@unicas.it (M.D.M.); francesca.dirocco@uniroma5.it (F.D.R.); silvia.zema@unicas.it (S.Z.)
2 European University of Technology EUt+, 03043 Cassino, Italy
3 Department of Human Sciences and Promotion of the Quality of Life, "San Raffaele" Open University of Rome, 00166 Rome, Italy
4 Department of Medicine and Aging Sciences, University "G. d'Annunzio" of Chieti-Pescara, 66100 Chieti, Italy; andrea.fusco@unich.it
* Correspondence: c.cortis@unicas.it

Highlights

What are the main findings?

- A single mini-trampoline training session decreased inter-limb asymmetry in participants with higher baseline inter-limb asymmetry, without affecting countermovement jump performance.
- Participants with lower baseline inter-limb asymmetry did not show a reduction in inter-limb asymmetry, showing a decrease in CMJ performance, possibly reflecting fatigue-related compensatory strategies.

What are the implications of the main findings?

- Mini-trampoline training may serve as an effective exercise to acutely reduce asymmetries in individuals at higher injury risk.
- Given its low impact, mini-trampoline training represents a safe and accessible plyometric exercise to use in preventive and rehabilitative programs.

Abstract

Background: Inter-limb asymmetry has implications for both athletic performance and healthcare practice. High baseline inter-limb asymmetries have been associated with impaired mobility, increased fall risk, and musculoskeletal injuries across the lifespan. Exercise interventions able to stimulate the stretch–shortening cycle (e.g., plyometric training and jump training) have been shown to have a good impact on asymmetries. Among these, Mini-Trampoline Training (MTT) has recently emerged as potentially effective in reducing asymmetries. **Objectives**: The study aimed to evaluate the acute effects of a single MTT session on muscle power and inter-limb asymmetry in young adults. **Methods**: Twenty-eight recreationally active participants (25.6 ± 2.4 years) completed one MTT session. Before (PRE) and after (POST) the MTT session, single-leg 6 m Timed Hop (6MTH) and countermovement jump (CMJ) tests were administered. Additionally, 6MTH values of the dominant (DOM) and non-dominant (NODOM) limbs were used to stratify participants according to higher (HBIA) or lower (LBIA) baseline inter-limb asymmetry, based on a commonly adopted Normalized Symmetry Index (NSI) threshold (NSI $\geq$ 10%, n = 12;

NSI < 10%, n = 16). Repeated-measures mixed models were used to evaluate the effects of the MTT session on 6MTH, NSI, and CMJ. **Results:** Regardless of group and limb, significant ($p < 0.0001$) improvements in 6MTH (PRE: 2.5 ± 0.06 s; POST: 2.3 ± 0.05 s) were found. Interestingly, the MTT session had a significant ($p = 0.01$) effect on both groups, with a significant ($p = 0.003$) interaction with NSI values, showing an improvement for HBIA (PRE = 15.4 ± 1.1%, POST = 11.3 ± 2.1%), whereas a decrement in LBIA was recorded (PRE = 5.1 ± 0.6%, POST = 9.6 ± 1.5%). CMJ did not show any changes in HBIA (PRE: 36.2 ± 0.9 cm; POST: 35.1 ± 0.7 cm), while a significant ($p = 0.007$) decrease was found in LBIA (PRE: 34.8 ± 1.2 cm; POST: 33.2 ± 1.3 cm). **Conclusions**: A single MTT session induced acute neuromuscular fatigue, reflected by reduced CMJ performance and improved (~8%) inter-limb control during hopping. The HBIA group preserved jump height (~36 cm) and demonstrated a significant reduction in asymmetry (NSI: −4.1%), suggesting more balanced lower-limb recruitment. Conversely, LBIA showed a significant decrease in CMJ and an increased NSI (+4.5%), possibly reflecting fatigue-related compensatory strategies. Overall, a single MTT elicited distinct responses according to baseline asymmetry, supporting its potential as an adaptable modality for enhancing neuromuscular function in HBIA.

Keywords: prevention; inter-limb asymmetry; health promotion; countermovement jump; plyometric

1. Introduction

Inter-limb asymmetry, or inter-limb difference, referring to the differences in function or performance between upper or lower limbs [1], is a relevant parameter in both athletic performance monitoring and healthcare practice [2]. Several methodologies to quantify asymmetries have been established as the difference between dominant and non-dominant [3], stronger and weaker [4], right and left [5] and injured and un-injured [6] limbs. Despite this variety of methodologies, no standardized method has been established, with the percentage difference between limbs remaining the most widely used approach [7].

Evidence [8–11] indicates that inter-limb asymmetry is prevalent among adolescents and elite athletes engaged in various sports (e.g., football, short track speed skating, volleyball, basketball, and karate) as a consequence of repeated unilateral or sport-specific motor patterns. A similar phenomenon is observed in non-athletic populations, such as older adults, where inter-limb asymmetry occurs due to age-related neuromuscular decline, sarcopenia, or neurological conditions (e.g., Parkinson's disease and Alzheimer's disease) [12]. Moreover, high baseline inter-limb asymmetry levels (≥10–15%) can compromise gait efficiency and increase fall risk [5,13]. Given their implications across both performance- and health-related domains, there is growing interest in interventions aimed at treating both participants with higher and lower baseline inter-limb asymmetries within sports and healthcare contexts.

The most effective non-pharmacological strategies for the treatment of inter-limb asymmetry are found in exercise-based interventions [14]. In particular, plyometric exercises have been shown to enhance neuromuscular function, improving performance and decreasing injury risk in both athletic and participants with higher baseline inter-limb asymmetry populations, through improvements in stretch–shortening cycle function, muscular strength, power, and coordination [14,15]. Among these activities, mini-trampoline training (MTT) represents a form of plyometric exercise combining aerobic and anaerobic demands with rhythmic and music-driven movements. In particular, MTT has been shown

https://doi.org/10.3390/healthcare14020160

to improve bone metabolism, body composition, balance, and neuromuscular coordination in different populations [16–18]. By reducing impact forces compared with traditional plyometric drills performed on rigid surfaces, MTT offers a safer and more accessible training modality. In addition, the compliant surface of the mini-trampoline allows the execution of repetitive plyometric actions with lower joint loading and mechanical stress, which may be particularly suitable for participants with higher baseline inter-limb asymmetry, balance deficits, or increased injury risk. These characteristics make MTT a promising alternative to traditional plyometric training in healthcare and preventive contexts. Despite its high potential, little is known about the acute effects of MTT on unilateral and bilateral functional lower-limb tasks.

Therefore, the present study aimed to examine the acute effects of a single MTT session on unilateral and bilateral jumping performance and inter-limb asymmetry in young adults with higher and lower baseline inter-limb asymmetry. We hypothesized that a single MTT session would acutely reduce asymmetry in participants with higher baseline inter-limb asymmetry, while not inducing clinically relevant increases in asymmetry in participants with lower baseline inter-limb asymmetry, thereby supporting its potential application in both health-related and injury-prevention contexts.

2. Materials and Methods

2.1. Experimental Approach to the Problem

This observational cohort study was conducted in accordance with the Declaration of Helsinki and the study protocol was approved on 4 December 2019 by the Institutional Review Board of the Department of Human Sciences, Society, and Health of the University of Cassino and Lazio Meridionale (approval number 26898) to evaluate the effects of the MTT on participants' Normalized Symmetry Index (NSI) and unilateral and bilateral jumping performance.

The 6 m Timed Hop (6MTH) test is widely adopted for the assessment of unilateral lower-limb performance and inter-limb asymmetry [19]. Given that both MTT and the 6MTH test involve repeated plyometric actions, examining the effects of MTT on 6MTH performance may help clarify its acute influence on neuromuscular function and asymmetry. Traditionally, inter-limb asymmetry in the 6MTH has been quantified using the Ratio Index, Symmetry Index, Symmetry Angle, or Gait Asymmetry [20]. However, these indices may produce non-linear results and perform asymptotically as values increase and do not provide a clear upper limit for asymmetry, which makes it difficult to interpret what should be considered a meaningful maximum value [20]. The NSI addresses these limitations by providing linear values, being normalized to variable magnitude and functioning as a bounded symmetry index. In the present study, the baseline NSI values were used to classify participants as those with higher baseline inter-limb asymmetry or lower baseline inter-limb asymmetry. Considering that MTT involves dynamic, elastic, and plyometric components relevant to lower-limb function and injury prevention, it could be interesting, in health contexts, to evaluate whether dynamic inter-limb asymmetries are influenced by a single session of MTT. Moreover, given that individuals with different baseline inter-limb asymmetry levels may respond differently to the training, this study also investigated the acute effects on unilateral hopping and vertical jump performance in individuals with higher and lower baseline inter-limb asymmetry.

To complement unilateral assessments, explosive performance was also evaluated through the Countermovement Jump (CMJ), a widely used measure of lower-limb power. The CMJ was included to provide additional information on global neuromuscular responses to MTT, particularly with respect to acute neuromuscular fatigue, given its sensitivity to short-term neuromuscular impairment [21,22]. Although the CMJ is performed

https://doi.org/10.3390/healthcare14020160

bilaterally and does not directly quantify inter-limb asymmetry, its jump height reflects the combined force and power output of both limbs and is sensitive to acute neuromuscular fatigue [23]. In this context, CMJ performance was used to help interpret whether changes observed in unilateral hopping and asymmetry indices occurred alongside signs of generalized fatigue or altered neuromuscular function following MTT.

The assessment of bilateral and unilateral jumping performance was completed before (PRE) and after (POST) MTT training. Baseline NSI values obtained at PRE were used exclusively for participant classification into higher (≥10%) and lower (<10%) baseline inter-limb asymmetry. Changes in NSI following the MTT session (POST–PRE) were then analyzed as outcome measures to evaluate acute modifications in inter-limb asymmetry. Thus, group classification and outcome assessment were based on temporally distinct measurements. In the absence of a non-exercise control condition, participants with lower baseline inter-limb asymmetry were included as a reference comparison group, allowing the examination of whether acute responses to MTT differed according to baseline asymmetry levels. This comparative approach was intended to distinguish changes potentially related to the training stimulus from those attributable to repeated testing or time-related effects, while acknowledging the observational nature of the study design. Additionally, to avoid the influence of fatigue on the evaluation, participants were asked to refrain from moderate-to-vigorous physical activity for 24 h before the experimental sessions.

2.2. Participants

Thirty-two (17 females and 15 males) recreationally active students voluntarily participated in this study and received information about the procedures and the aim of the study. All participants were asked to read and sign the consent form, and they were able to withdraw from the study at any time for any reason, without any consequences. Participants with prior experience in MTT and those who reported preexisting limitations such as cardiovascular, respiratory, metabolic diseases, and musculoskeletal injuries of the back or lower extremities were excluded from the study. Participants were classified as recreationally active and included in the study if they reported participating in at least 150 to 300 min of moderate-intensity exercise or 75 to 150 min of vigorous-intensity exercise per week, plus muscle-strengthening activities 2 or more days per week, over the previous 6 months [24,25]. These criteria were used to exclude sedentary individuals and frequent MTT users and were not intended to provide a detailed quantification of habitual physical activity levels or exercise intensity. In accordance with Regulation (EU) 2016/679, to maintain anonymity, each participant was assigned a unique identification code, and personal data were solely used for statistical purposes.

2.3. Procedures

Before starting the testing session, individuals' anthropometric measures were collected. Height and body mass were measured to the nearest 0.1 cm and 0.1 kg, respectively, by using a scale with an integrated stadiometer (Seca 709, Vogel & Halke, Hamburg, Germany). Body mass index (BMI) was subsequently calculated and reported as weight (kg)/height (m^2). Preferred dominant lower limb was determined using a functional task, defined as the limb spontaneously used when stepping on a platform, in accordance with the previous literature [18,26].

2.4. Mini-Trampoline Training

MTT session was performed on a mini-trampoline (CoalSport, Rome, Italy) with the diameter of the elastic surface of 122 cm. The MTT included a session of free practice on the mini-trampoline and 30 min of workout. During the warm-up (5 min) and cool down (5 min) phases, participants were required to continuously jump on the mini-trampoline

 https://doi.org/10.3390/healthcare14020160

while performing breathing and mobility exercises. The central phase (20 min) consisted of jumping exercises, including single and double hops on different planes, and jumping jacks, double hops with wide and close stances, performed in combination with movements of the upper body. The total duration for the session was ~40 min [27].

2.5. 6 m Timed Hop

The 6MTH test involved multiple consecutive single limb hops on the same limb over a distance of 6 m. A 6 m long, 15 cm wide line was marked on the floor with a standard tape measure placed along the middle, perpendicular to the starting line. Before the tests, participants performed a standardized warm-up of 5 min at low resistance on an upright bike at a self-determined intensity, followed by mobility exercise for the lower limb. After warm-up, all participants completed a familiarization phase of 3 practice trials of 6MTH, to ensure correct understanding of the test procedures and reduce potential learning effects [24]. Following the practice trials, participants performed one testing trial of the 6MTH per limb. Participants stood on one limb (dominant or non-dominant) with their toes aligned at the starting line and began hopping upon the verbal '3-2-1' countdown given by the principal investigator. Participants were instructed to hop over the designated distance in as little time as possible and then gradually slow down to a stop, after which they were asked to walk back to the starting line at a comfortable pace. The test ended when the heel of the tested limb crossed the finish line. Both limbs were tested in random order, and no restrictions were given to participants regarding arm movement. A rest period of 30 s was given between limbs. The time taken to cross the 6 m distance was recorded in seconds using a handheld stopwatch (Seiko Stopwatch, Soler Standard SVAJ001) capable of measuring to the 1/100th of a second and recording multiple split times. The stopwatch was operated by a certified Italian Timekeepers Federation operator, trained in manual timing procedures and movement analysis techniques. Measurements were recorded to the nearest 100th of a second.

2.6. Normalized Symmetry Index

The NSI was used to assess symmetry between the dominant and non-dominant limb, calculated as follows [20]:

$$\frac{(\mathrm{ndl} - \mathrm{dl})}{\max = (0, \mathrm{ndl}, \mathrm{dl}) - \min = (0, \mathrm{ndl}, \mathrm{dl})} \cdot 100 \tag{1}$$

where ndl = non-dominant limb, dl = dominant limb, max = highest value between non-dominant and dominant, and min = lowest value between non-dominant and dominant.

In this formula, the numerator represents the difference between the non-dominant and dominant limb. The denominator represents the maximum and minimum values for the measure across the trial. Given that the values of 6MTH performance are positive, 0 was used as the minimum value. The NSI provides a normalized percentage of asymmetry, where a value of 0% indicates perfect symmetry and a maximum value of 100% indicates maximum asymmetry between limbs. As proposed by previous studies [28,29], an asymmetry threshold of $\geq$10%, indicative of a higher risk of injury, was used to classify participants as having higher baseline inter-limb asymmetry.

From a total of thirty-two participants who began the study, four were excluded due to not meeting the inclusion criteria. Subsequently, the twenty-eight subjects were allocated into two groups, according to their baseline asymmetry values. The number of participants with higher baseline inter-limb asymmetry was 12, while the number of participants with lower baseline inter-limb asymmetry was 16 (Figure 1). All participants

 https://doi.org/10.3390/healthcare14020160

were healthy young adults, with the ≥10% NSI threshold being used exclusively for baseline stratification purposes and not indicating a clinical diagnosis.

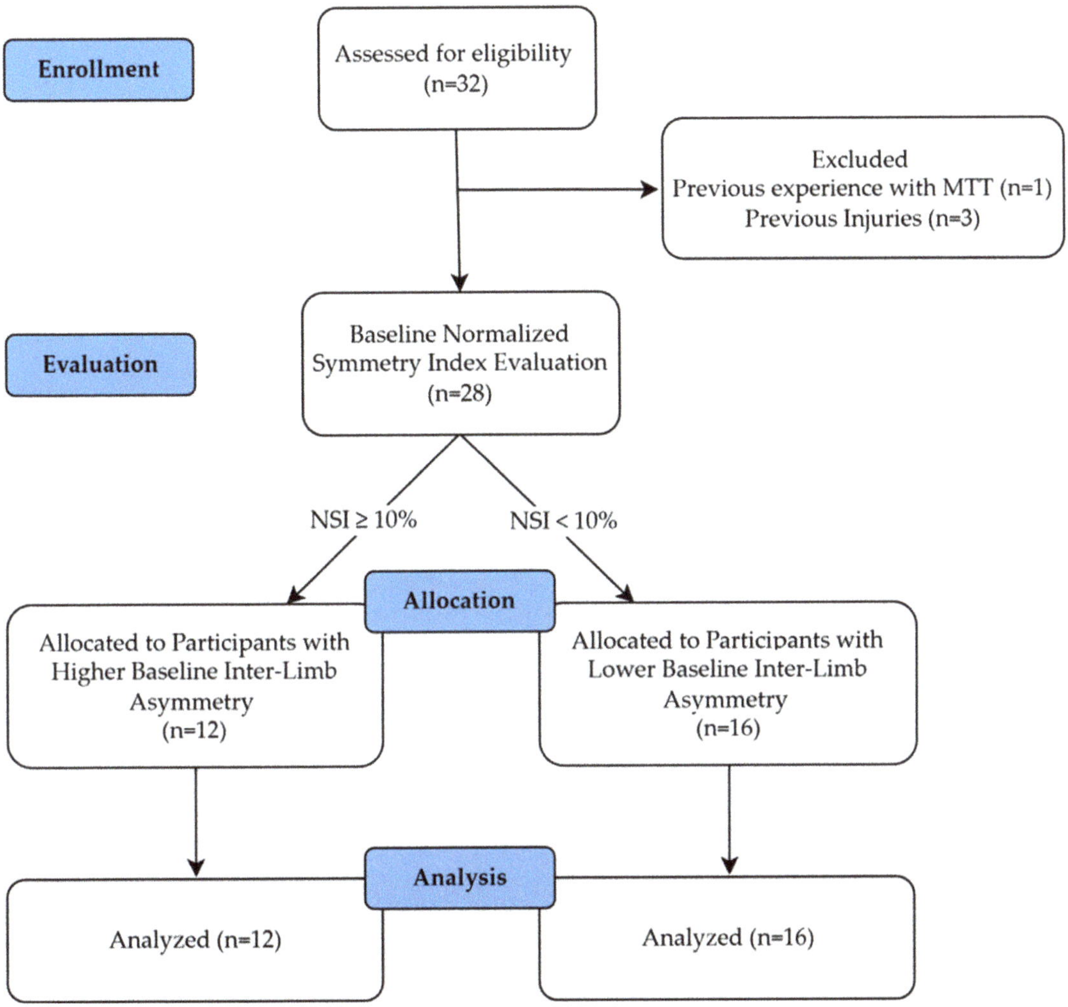

Figure 1. Flow chart of the recruitment and selection process of the subjects included in the study. MTT: Mini-Trampoline Training; NSI: Normalized Symmetry Index.

2.7. Countermovement Jump

Participants were instructed to stand with their feet shoulder-width apart to perform a fast downward movement to approximately 90° of flexion at the hip and knee, immediately followed by an upward movement. Participants were asked to jump as high as possible, keeping their hands on their hips, to make their trunk as upright as possible throughout the entire jump, and land with their legs fully extended. To familiarize the participants with the jumping technique, a number (3 to 5) of submaximal jumps were conducted before data collection. Subsequently, participants performed three jumps, with a 1 min recovery between attempts, and the best was used for analysis. This approach was adopted to reduce the potential impact of confounding factors such as neuromuscular fatigue and fluctuations in performance related to circadian rhythms, both of which can affect motor output and

https://doi.org/10.3390/healthcare14020160

measurement reliability. CMJ performance was recorded using the Quattro Jump 9290BA force plate (Kistler, Winterthur, Switzerland). Data were recorded at a sampling frequency of 500 Hz. The force plate calculated the time between the take-off and landing phases, used to establish jump heights [30].

2.8. Statistical Analysis

STATA software version 18 (StataCorp, College Station, TX, USA) was used for statistical analysis. Means, standard deviations (SD) and 95% confidence intervals (95% CI) were calculated for all variables. The Shapiro–Wilk test was used to assess the normal distribution of the data. Linear repeated-measures mixed model analyses were performed to examine the effects of the MTT on individuals' 6MTH, NSI, and CMJ performance. Linear repeated-measures mixed model analyses were intentionally chosen because they account for individual variability and are more robust to violations of sphericity [31]. Effect Size (d, η_p^2) was calculated to determine the magnitude of the effects. Cohen's d was interpreted as trivial (<0.2), small (0.2 to 0.6), moderate (0.61 to 1.2), or large (>1.2), and η_p^2 was interpreted as 0.01 (small), 0.06 (medium), and 0.14 (large) [32]. For these analyses, the level of significance was set at $p < 0.05$. Because baseline NSI was used for stratification, inferential interpretation focused on PRE–POST changes in NSI and the time × baseline asymmetry interaction, rather than on baseline group differences, which were expected by design. Moreover, because the asymmetry classification (≥10% NSI) was derived from baseline NSI values and could be influenced by regression to the mean, a sensitivity analysis was performed to avoid dichotomization. Specifically, baseline NSI (PRE) was calculated for each participant and included as a continuous moderator in a repeated-measures mixed-effects model testing the time × baseline NSI interaction (PRE vs. POST). Model estimation was performed using restricted maximum likelihood with the subject specified as a random effect.

3. Results

The anthropometric characteristics of the participants, divided by baseline NSI values, are presented in Table 1.

Table 1. Mean values and standard deviations of the participants' characteristics.

	Participants with Lower Baseline Inter-Limb Asymmetry	Participants with Higher Baseline Inter-Limb Asymmetry	Total
N	16	12	28
Age (years)	24.3 ± 1.2	27.2 ± 2.8	25.6 ± 2.4
Body height (m)	1.59 ± 0.0	1.74 ± 0.1	1.65 ± 0.1
Body mass (kg)	56.6 ± 5.7	72.7 ± 11.9	63.5 ± 11.9
BMI (kg·m^{-2})	22.4 ± 2.3	24.0 ± 3.2	23.1 ± 2.5

N = Number; BMI = Body Mass Index.

The analysis showed a significant main effect of time ($F_{(1,83)}$ = 5.82, p = 0.01, η_p^2 = 0.09), indicating a difference in 6MTH performance between PRE (d = 0.21; dominant: 2.46 ± 0.48 s; non-dominant: 2.51 ± 0.41 s) and POST (d = 0.27; dominant: 2.36 ± 0.44 s; non-dominant: 2.38 ± 0.44 s) MTT session regardless of group and limb (Supplementary Figure S1).

The model was found to be statistically significant for NSI (Supplementary Figure S2; $F_{(1,26)}$ = 8.94, p = 0.0003), with a significant main effect found for time (p < 0.001, 95%CI: 6.21 to 14.51) and group (p = 0.01, 95%CI: 1.09 to 8.23), and a significant interaction (p = 0.003,

https://doi.org/10.3390/healthcare14020160

95%CI: −14.11 to −3.21). Specifically, NSI values were different between PRE and POST in both participants with higher baseline inter-limb asymmetry (*d* = 0.69; PRE: 15.4 ± 3.8%; POST: 11.3 ± 7.4%) and participants with lower baseline inter-limb asymmetry (*d* = 0.99; PRE: 5.0 ± 2.7%; POST: 9.7 ± 6.1%) populations. Additionally, PRE values were significantly different among groups (*d* = 3.1; $p < 0.001$, 95%CI: 6.39 to 14.32); thus, the difference did not persist in POST evaluation ($p = 0.4$, 95%CI: −2.26 to 5.65). Additionally, a significant time × baseline NSI interaction was observed (β = −0.78, SE = 0.21, $p < 0.001$), indicating that both the magnitude and the direction of PRE–POST changes in asymmetry depended on baseline NSI values.

Lastly, CMJ analysis showed the significance of the model ($F_{(3,26)} = 3.39$, $p = 0.003$, $\eta_p^2 = 0.28$), with a significant main effect found for time ($p = 0.01$, 95%CI: −2.88 to −0.35). Specifically, in participants with lower baseline inter-limb asymmetry, significant (*d* = 1.27; $p = 0.009$; 95%CI: −2.82 to −0.41) differences emerged between PRE (34.8 ± 1.2 cm) and POST (33.2 ± 1.3 cm) evaluation. No significant interactions were detected.

Means, SD, contrast, 95% CI, and interaction effects of all variables are shown in Table 2.

Table 2. Means, standard deviations (SD), contrast, 95% confidence intervals (95% CI), and interaction effects of the 6 m Timed Hop Test (6MTH), Normalized Symmetry Index, and Countermovement Jump Test before and after the mini-trampoline training session.

		PRE	POST		Interactions
		Mean ± SD	Mean ± SD	Contrast (95%CI)	Time × Group
Participants with Higher Baseline Inter-Limb Asymmetry (n = 12)	6MTH in Dominant limb (s)	2.37 ± 0.59	2.37 ± 0.49	0.06 (−0.25 to 0.11)	$p = 0.46$
	6MTH in Non-dominant limb (s)	2.54 ± 0.39	2.33 ± 0.32	0.21 (−0.41 to −0.01)	$p = 0.03$
	Normalized Symmetry Index (%)	15.38 ± 3.81	11.38 ± 3.24	4.00 (−7.92 to −0.07)	$p = 0.04$
	Countermovement Jump (cm)	36.24 ± 3.24	35.17 ± 2.74	1.07 (−2.46 to 0.32)	$p = 0.13$
		PRE	POST		Interactions
		Mean ± SD	Mean ± SD	Contrast (95%CI)	Time × Group
Participants with Lower Baseline Inter-Limb Asymmetry (n = 16)	6MTH in Dominant limb (s)	2.53 ± 0.47	2.42 ± 0.44	0.11 (−0.27 to 0.04)	$p = 0.16$
	6MTH in Non-dominant limb (s)	2.48 ± 0.44	2.42 ± 0.52	0.06 (−0.23 to 0.11)	$p = 0.46$
	Normalized Symmetry Index (%)	5.02 ± 2.72	9.69 ± 6.12	4.66 (1.26 to 8.06)	$p = 0.007$
	Countermovement Jump (cm)	34.88 ± 4.93	33.26 ± 5.53	1.61 (−2.82 to −0.41)	$p = 0.009$

4. Discussion

This study examined the acute effects of a single MTT session on unilateral and vertical jump performance and inter-limb asymmetry. Our findings showed a significant interaction between time (PRE vs. POST) and group (participants with higher vs. participants with lower baseline inter-limb asymmetry), whereby participants with higher baseline inter-limb asymmetry levels demonstrated a decrease in NSI (–4.0%) after MTT, whereas those with lower baseline inter-limb asymmetry levels showed a small, non-significant increase (4.6%), which remained below the critical cut-off. Although we hypothesized that asymmetry would remain stable in participants with lower baseline inter-limb asymmetry, the small increase observed following MTT should not be interpreted as a negative or clinically relevant outcome. Rather, it likely reflects a transient acute response to the training stimulus, potentially driven by post-session neuromuscular fatigue or short-term compensatory motor strategies adopted during post-intervention testing. Regarding 6MTH performance, participants completed the test faster after MTT, regardless of the limb used and the group, indicating an acute improvement in lower-limb functional performance.

Repetitive jumping on a mini-trampoline involves stretch–shortening cycle actions comparable to traditional plyometric training, but with reduced mechanical load due to the compliant surface [15,33]. Previous studies [18,27] have shown that MTT can enhance balance and leg stiffness, supporting its potential application in both preventive and re-

 https://doi.org/10.3390/healthcare14020160

habilitative contexts. Specifically, Di Rocco et al. [27] showed that, despite the elastic and compliant nature of the mini-trampoline surface, a single session induced a reduction in reactive power, interpreted as an acute neuromuscular fatigue response. In contrast, leg stiffness did not change, indicating that MTT might exert a protective effect on leg stiffness, preventing acute decreases that are commonly observed in other training modalities. Consistent with these findings, our results suggest that even a single session may help reduce inter-limb asymmetry in individuals with higher baseline values. The contrasting responses between groups can be explained by their different baseline asymmetry values. These group differences align with the concept of baseline dependency, in which individuals with greater initial asymmetry typically show larger acute improvements, a pattern also documented in previous plyometric training studies [18]. This reinforces that baseline asymmetry is a key factor influencing the magnitude of acute adaptations. Regarding vertical jump performance, CMJ performance decreased only in participants with lower baseline inter-limb asymmetry. This reduction may be attributed to acute neuromuscular fatigue associated with plyometric exercise, involving mechanical, neuromuscular, and metabolic factors [34]. The lack of decrease in the participants with higher baseline inter-limb asymmetry may indicate a more balanced force and power contribution from both limbs following the intervention. However, this remains speculative and cannot be confirmed without direct biomechanical measures. It should be noted that CMJ performance was not intended to assess inter-limb asymmetry per se, but rather to contextualize unilateral performance outcomes within a measure of overall bilateral neuromuscular function. The improvement observed in 6MTH performance, combined with the reduction or stability in CMJ performance, could also be related to the specific demands of the training. MTT primarily involves repeated bilateral jumps that more closely resemble the 6MTH task than the CMJ, possibly facilitating better neuromuscular activation patterns for hopping performance. A mild post-activation potentiation effect cannot be excluded, but should be considered only as a possible contributing factor, given that CMJ performance did not improve uniformly [35].

Overall, these findings indicate that MTT may acutely benefit individuals with higher baseline inter-limb asymmetry, while inducing a fatigue-related response in those with minimal asymmetry. This highlights how the same training stimulus may yield different short-term outcomes depending on initial functional status. From a healthcare perspective, these results have important implications as inter-limb asymmetry has been associated with increased musculoskeletal injury risk and reduced functional mobility [36]. In this context, the present findings support the potential role of MTT primarily in clinical and rehabilitative contexts, particularly for participants with higher baseline inter-limb asymmetry. The reduced impact forces of the mini-trampoline limit landing stress and may lower injury risk, making this modality suitable for populations with joint instability or balance deficits. Additionally, the accessibility and enjoyable nature of MTT may enhance long-term adherence to exercise interventions, which is essential for promoting sustained health benefits [37].

5. Conclusions

This study demonstrated that a single MTT session can acutely reduce inter-limb asymmetry, depending on baseline asymmetry values, during unilateral hopping without affecting CMJ performance in participants with higher baseline inter-limb asymmetry. Participants with higher baseline inter-limb asymmetry showed a reduction in NSI after MTT, compared to the participants with lower baseline inter-limb asymmetry, confirming that individuals with a higher level of asymmetry may achieve greater benefits in reducing performance imbalance during the 6MTH. From a practical perspective, mini-trampoline

https://doi.org/10.3390/healthcare14020160

exercise represents an accessible and safe intervention that may be particularly beneficial within clinical and rehabilitative programs aimed at reducing functional inter-limb asymmetry in individuals with higher baseline asymmetry. Future research should investigate the long-term effects of MTT and evaluate its applicability in several populations, including sedentary adults, older individuals, and participants with higher baseline inter-limb asymmetry. Additionally, the use of automated measurement tools, such as timing gates or photocells, should be considered to enhance accuracy and reduce potential measurement error. Confirming its effectiveness across different settings could establish MTT as a valuable non-pharmacological intervention to improve functional capacity, prevent injury, and promote health and well-being across the lifespan.

6. Limitations

This study has several limitations that must be acknowledged when interpreting the findings. These include a relatively small sample size restricted to healthy young adults, the short term evaluation, and the absence of a non-exercise control group, which limits generalizability to clinical or older populations. Although participants with lower baseline inter-limb asymmetry were included as a reference comparison group to explore differential acute responses to MTT, this approach does not fully account for potential learning, fatigue, or time-related effects. Additionally, the study examined the short-term effects of a single session of MTT. Consequently, the present findings are specific to the acute response to exercise, whereas potential long-term effects necessitate further investigations. Using the 6MTH test to assess asymmetry may not capture all aspects of functional imbalance. Therefore, additional tests such as single hop, triple hop, and crossover hop could be considered for inclusion in future studies to better capture functional asymmetry. In addition, the lack of detailed biomechanical data (e.g., limb-specific force output or force symmetry during jumping tasks) limits the ability to explain the neuromuscular mechanisms underlying the preserved CMJ performance observed in participants with higher baseline inter-limb asymmetry.

Supplementary Materials: The following supporting information can be downloaded at https://www.mdpi.com/article/10.3390/healthcare14020160/s1. Figure S1. Distribution of 6 m Timed Hop Test performance before (PRE) and after (POST) the mini-trampoline intervention for the dominant and non-dominant limb. The 6MTH performance was significantly ($p = 0.01$) different between PRE and POST MTT session regardless of group and limb. Figure S2. Distribution of the Normalized Symmetry Index before (PRE) and after (POST) the mini-trampoline intervention in both groups. * Significantly ($p = 0.01$) different between PRE and POST in both groups. # PRE values significantly ($p < 0.001$) different among groups; thus, the difference did not persist in the POST evaluation

Author Contributions: Conceptualization, C.C. and A.F.; data curation, O.P.; formal analysis, O.P.; funding acquisition, C.C.; investigation, M.D.M. and A.F.; methodology, C.C. and A.F.; project administration, C.C.; supervision, C.C. and A.F.; writing—original draft, O.P., E.F., M.D.M., F.D.R., S.Z., C.C. and A.F.; writing—review and editing, O.P., E.F., M.D.M., F.D.R., S.Z., C.C. and A.F. All authors have read and agreed to the published version of the manuscript.

Funding: This research received no external funding.

Institutional Review Board Statement: The study was conducted in accordance with the Declaration of Helsinki and approved by the Institutional Review Board of the University of Cassino and Lazio Meridionale (approval number 26898; approval date: 4 December 2019).

Informed Consent Statement: Written informed consent was obtained from the patients to publish this paper.

https://doi.org/10.3390/healthcare14020160

Data Availability Statement: The original data presented in the study are openly available at https://github.com/ccortis/DataHop.git.

Conflicts of Interest: The authors declare no conflicts of interest.

Abbreviations

The following abbreviations are used in this manuscript:

MTT	Mini-Trampoline Training
6MTH	6 m Timed Hop
CMJ	Countermovement Jump
NSI	Normalized Symmetry Index
N	Number
BMI	Body Mass Index
SD	Standard Deviation
CI	Confidence Interval
dl	Dominant Limb
ndl	Non-Dominant Limb

References

1. Espada, M.C.; Jardim, M.; Assunção, R.; Estaca, A.; Ferreira, C.C.; Pessôa Filho, D.M.; Verardi, C.E.L.; Gamonales, J.M.; Santos, F.J. Lower Limb Unilateral and Bilateral Strength Asymmetry in High-Level Male Senior and Professional Football Players. *Healthcare* **2023**, *11*, 1579. [CrossRef] [PubMed]
2. Afonso, J.; Virgile, A.; Peña, J.; Jordan, M.; García-de-Alcaraz, A.; Sá, M.; Bishop, C. On Uneven Ground: Embracing the Challenges of Inter-Limb Asymmetries and Their Assessment. *Asymmetry* **2025**, *1*, 4. [CrossRef]
3. Newton, R.U.; Gerber, A.; Nimphius, S.; Shim, J.K.; Doan, B.K.; Robertson, M.; Pearson, D.R.; Craig, B.W.; Häkkinen, K.; Kraemer, W.J. Determination of Functional Strength Imbalance of the Lower Extremities. *J. Strength Cond. Res.* **2006**, *20*, 971–977. [CrossRef] [PubMed]
4. Impellizzeri, F.M.; Rampinini, E.; Maffiuletti, N.; Marcora, S.M. A Vertical Jump Force Test for Assessing Bilateral Strength Asymmetry in Athletes. *Med. Sci. Sports Exerc.* **2007**, *39*, 2044–2050. [CrossRef]
5. Sun, W.; Li, H.; Qu, L.; Zhou, Y.; Cao, X.; Wang, K.; Li, K. Unilateral Plyometric Training Effectively Reduces Lower Limb Asymmetry in Athletes: A Meta-Analysis. *Front. Physiol.* **2025**, *16*, 1551523. [CrossRef]
6. Ardern, C.L.; Webster, K.E.; Taylor, N.F.; Feller, J.A. Return to the Preinjury Level of Competitive Sport After Anterior Cruciate Ligament Reconstruction Surgery. *Am. J. Sports Med.* **2011**, *39*, 538–543. [CrossRef]
7. Bishop, C.; Turner, A.; Read, P. Effects of Inter-Limb Asymmetries on Physical and Sports Performance: A Systematic Review. *J. Sports Sci.* **2018**, *36*, 1135–1144. [CrossRef]
8. Śliwowski, R.; Paillard, T.; Bojkowski, Ł.; Dudziński, W.; Patek, M.; Marynowicz, J. Intra- and Inter-Limb Strength Imbalance and Asymmetry in Soccer: A Comparison of Elite Senior and Junior Players. *PLoS ONE* **2024**, *19*, e0302474. [CrossRef]
9. Kalata, M.; Williams, C.A.; Verbruggen, F.F.; De Ste Croix, M.; Lehnert, M.; Zahalka, F.; Maly, T. Strength and Jumping Performance in Youth Athletes: Do Sport Specialization and Age Categories Affect Strength Asymmetry? *Res. Sport Med.* **2025**, *33*, 334–351. [CrossRef]
10. Ojeda-Aravena, A.; Warnier-Medina, A.; Brand, C.; Morales-Zúñiga, J.; Orellana-Lepe, G.; Zapata-Bastias, J.; Tuesta, M. Relationship between Body Composition Asymmetry and Specific Performance in Taekwondo Athletes: A Cross-Sectional Study. *Symmetry* **2023**, *15*, 2087. [CrossRef]
11. Gaweł, E.; Drozd, M.; Maszczyk, A.; Zając, A. Acute Effects of a Simulated Karate Bout on Muscular Strength Asymmetries of the Lower Limbs in Elite Athletes of Different Age Categories. *Appl. Sci.* **2025**, *15*, 888. [CrossRef]
12. Perry, M.C.; Carville, S.F.; Smith, I.C.H.; Rutherford, O.M.; Newham, D.J. Strength, Power Output and Symmetry of Leg Muscles: Effect of Age and History of Falling. *Eur. J. Appl. Physiol.* **2007**, *100*, 553–561. [CrossRef] [PubMed]
13. Klawitter, L.; Bradley, A.; Hackney, K.; Tomkinson, G.; Christensen, B.; Kraemer, W.; McGrath, R. The Associations between Asymmetric Handgrip Strength and Chronic Disease Status in American Adults: Results from the National Health and Nutrition Examination Survey. *J. Funct. Morphol. Kinesiol.* **2021**, *6*, 79. [CrossRef] [PubMed]
14. Ramírez-Campillo, R.; Andrade, D.C.; Izquierdo, M. Effects of Plyometric Training Volume and Training Surface on Explosive Strength. *J. Strength Cond. Res.* **2013**, *27*, 2714–2722. [CrossRef]
15. Sáez-Sáez de Villarreal, E.; Requena, B.; Newton, R.U. Does Plyometric Training Improve Strength Performance? A Meta-Analysis. *J. Sci. Med. Sport* **2010**, *13*, 513–522. [CrossRef]

https://doi.org/10.3390/healthcare14020160

16. Vasto, S.; Amato, A.; Proia, P.; Caldarella, R.; Cortis, C.; Baldassano, S. Dare to Jump: The Effect of the New High Impact Activity SuperJump on Bone Remodeling. A New Tool to Maintain Fitness during COVID-19 Home Confinement. *Biol. Sport* **2022**, *39*, 1011–1019. [CrossRef]
17. Contrò, V.; Bianco, A.; Cooper, J.; Sacco, A.; Macchiarella, A.; Traina, M.; Proia, P. Effects of Different Circuit Training Protocols on Body Mass, Fat Mass and Blood Parameters in Overweight Adults. *J. Biol. Res. Boll. Della Soc. Ital. Di Biol. Sper.* **2017**, *90*, 6279. [CrossRef]
18. De Maio, M.; Di Rocco, F.; Papale, O.; Festino, E.; Fusco, A.; Cortis, C. Could Mini-Trampoline Training Be Considered as a New Strategy to Reduce Asymmetries? *Appl. Sci.* **2023**, *13*, 3193. [CrossRef]
19. Ebert, J.R.; Du Preez, L.; Furzer, B.; Edwards, P.; Joss, B. Which Hop Tests Can Best Identify Functional Limb Asymmetry in Patients 9–12 Months After Anterior Cruciate Ligament Reconstruction Employing a Hamstrings Tendon Autograft? *Int. J. Sports Phys. Ther.* **2021**, *16*, 393–403. [CrossRef]
20. Queen, R.; Dickerson, L.; Ranganathan, S.; Schmitt, D. A Novel Method for Measuring Asymmetry in Kinematic and Kinetic Variables: The Normalized Symmetry Index. *J. Biomech.* **2020**, *99*, 109531. [CrossRef]
21. Markovic, G.; Dizdar, D.; Jukic, I.; Cardinale, M. Reliability and Factorial Validity of Squat and Countermovement Jump Tests. *J. Strength Cond. Res.* **2004**, *18*, 551–555.
22. Stockbrugger, B.A.; Haennel, R.G. Contributing Factors to Performance of a Medicine Ball Explosive Power Test: A Comparison Between Jump and Nonjump Athletes. *J. Strength Cond. Res.* **2003**, *17*, 768–774. [CrossRef] [PubMed]
23. Cortis, C.; Tessitore, A.; Lupo, C.; Perroni, F.; Pesce, C.; Capranica, L. Changes in Jump, Sprint, and Coordinative Performances After a Senior Soccer Match. *J. Strength Cond. Res.* **2013**, *27*, 2989–2996. [CrossRef] [PubMed]
24. Munro, A.G.; Herrington, L.C. Between-Session Reliability of Four Hop Tests and the Agility T-Test. *J. Strength Cond. Res.* **2011**, *25*, 1470–1477. [CrossRef] [PubMed]
25. McKay, A.K.A.; Stellingwerff, T.; Smith, E.S.; Martin, D.T.; Mujika, I.; Goosey-Tolfrey, V.L.; Sheppard, J.; Burke, L.M. Defining Training and Performance Caliber: A Participant Classification Framework. *Int. J. Sports Physiol. Perform.* **2022**, *17*, 317–331. [CrossRef]
26. Steidl-Müller, L.; Hildebrandt, C.; Müller, E.; Fink, C.; Raschner, C. Limb Symmetry Index in Competitive Alpine Ski Racers: Reference Values and Injury Risk Identification According to Age-Related Performance Levels. *J. Sport Health Sci.* **2018**, *7*, 405–415. [CrossRef]
27. Di Rocco, F.; Papale, O.; Festino, E.; De Maio, M.; Cortis, C.; Fusco, A. Acute Effects of Mini Trampoline Training Session on Leg Stiffness and Reactive Power. *Appl. Sci.* **2023**, *13*, 9865. [CrossRef]
28. Bishop, C. Interlimb Asymmetries: Are Thresholds a Usable Concept? *Strength Cond. J.* **2021**, *43*, 32–36. [CrossRef]
29. Philipp, N.M.; Crawford, D.A.; Garver, M.J.; Davis, D.W.; Hair, J. Interlimb Asymmetry Thresholds That Negatively Affect Change of Direction Performance in Collegiate American Football Players. *Int. J. Exerc. Sci.* **2021**, *14*, 606–612. [CrossRef]
30. Picerno, P.; Camomilla, V.; Capranica, L. Countermovement Jump Performance Assessment Using a Wearable 3D Inertial Measurement Unit. *J. Sports Sci.* **2011**, *29*, 139–146. [CrossRef]
31. van Wely, M. Mixed Models for Repetitive Measurements: The Basics. *Fertil. Steril.* **2024**, *121*, 914–917. [CrossRef]
32. Hopkins, W.G.; Marshall, S.W.; Battheram, A.M.; Hanin, J. Progressive Statistics for Studies in Sports Medicine and Exercise Science. *Med. Sci. Sports Exerc.* **2009**, *41*, 3–12. [CrossRef]
33. Booth, M.A.; Orr, R. Effects of Plyometric Training on Sports Performance. *Strength Cond. J.* **2016**, *38*, 30–37. [CrossRef]
34. Wu, P.P.-Y.; Sterkenburg, N.; Everett, K.; Chapman, D.W.; White, N.; Mengersen, K. Predicting Fatigue Using Countermovement Jump Force-Time Signatures: PCA Can Distinguish Neuromuscular versus Metabolic Fatigue. *PLoS ONE* **2019**, *14*, e0219295. [CrossRef]
35. Hodgson, M.; Docherty, D.; Robbins, D. Post-Activation Potentiation. *Sports Med.* **2005**, *35*, 585–595. [CrossRef]
36. Guan, Y.; Bredin, S.; Taunton, J.; Jiang, Q.; Wu, N.; Warburton, D. Association between Inter-Limb Asymmetries in Lower-Limb Functional Performance and Sport Injury: A Systematic Review of Prospective Cohort Studies. *J. Clin. Med.* **2022**, *11*, 360. [CrossRef]
37. Papale, O.; Festino, E.; Di Rocco, F.; Foster, C.; Prestanti, I.; Serafini, S.; Izzicupo, P.; Cortis, C.; Fusco, A. The Impact of a Multidimensional Physical Activity Intervention on Glycemic Control in Type 1 Diabetes: A Preliminary Study. *J. Funct. Morphol. Kinesiol.* **2025**, *10*, 163. [CrossRef]

 https://doi.org/10.3390/healthcare14020160

healthcare

MDPI

Article

Evaluating the Agreement and Associations with Physical Function Between Equation- and Linear Position Transducer-Estimated Sit-to-Stand Muscle Power in Aging Adults

Garrett Steinbrink *, Taylor Danielson, Julian Martinez, Joseph Patnode, Ann Swartz and Scott Strath *

Zilber College of Public Health, University of Wisconsin-Milwaukee, Milwaukee, WI 53211, USA; danie326@uwm.edu (T.D.); marti994@uwm.edu (J.M.); patnode@uwm.edu (J.P.); aswartz@uwm.edu (A.S.)
* Correspondence: garrett-steinbrink@uiowa.edu (G.S.); sstrath@uwm.edu (S.S.)

Abstract: Background/Objectives: Muscle power, estimated from the sit-to-stand (STS) test, is an important indicator of physical function (PF) in aging adults. Therefore, its assessment may be implemented into future clinical practice. The agreement between different STS power assessments is unknown, and the associations between methods and PF outcomes have not been compared. **Methods**: A total of 49 aging adults (mean age = 60.9 ± 10.9; 67% female) participated in this cross-sectional study. STS power from a validated equation (EQ) and a linear position transducer (LPT) were estimated. Handgrip strength (HGS), timed up-and-go (TUG), usual gait speed (UGS), fast gait speed (FGS), the 400-m walk test (400MWT), and self-reported total, basic lower-body, and advanced lower-body PF were assessed. The agreement of STS power methods was assessed with an intraclass correlation coefficient (ICC) and a Bland–Altman plot. Multiple linear regression evaluated the associations between STS power and PF outcomes. **Results**: EQ and LPT STS power demonstrated only moderate agreement (ICC = 0.69). EQ STS power was independently associated with TUG ($\beta = -0.45$), UGS ($\beta = 0.37$), FGS ($\beta = 0.48$), 400MWT ($\beta = -0.55$), self-reported total ($\beta = 0.30$), basic lower-body ($\beta = 0.30$), and advanced lower-body PF ($\beta = 0.30$), but not HGS ($\beta = 0.14$). LPT STS power was independently associated with HGS ($\beta = 0.44$), FGS ($\beta = 0.40$), 400MWT ($\beta = -0.51$), self-reported total ($\beta = 0.31$), basic lower-body ($\beta = 0.29$), and advanced lower-body PF ($\beta = 0.32$), but neither TUG ($\beta = -0.26$) nor UGS ($\beta = 0.28$). **Conclusions**: EQ and LPT STS power demonstrate limited agreement, and EQ STS power may be a superior indicator of PF in aging adults. Future research should examine the feasibility of implementing STS power tests in clinical settings to screen and refer patients with low muscle power to effective therapeutic interventions.

Keywords: strength; exercise; resistance training; older adults; physical activity; sarcopenia; frailty; primary care; gerontology

1. Introduction

Muscle power is an important indicator of physical function (PF), mobility, and mortality in aging adults [1,2]. Muscle power is a stronger predictor of gait performance, functional mobility, and falls in aging adults compared to muscle strength [3–7]. Additionally, muscle power significantly predicts all-cause mortality, irrespective of sedentary behavior, physical activity, and adiposity [8], suggesting it should be treated as a critical marker of healthy aging and longevity [9]. As the number of adults 65+ years of age is expected to double in the coming decades, the frequent and accurate assessment of muscle power may play an important role in routine clinical practice.

One of the limitations in assessing muscle power is the accessibility of valid, easy-to-implement, and safe measurement methods [1]. The most commonly used instrument to quantify muscle power in aging adults is the pneumatic leg press, which is largely infeasible for the clinical setting [10]. Due to these methodological limitations, various research groups have developed equations (EQs) to estimate muscle power from the sit-to-stand (STS) test [1,11]. Of the available EQs, the EQ developed by Alcazar and colleagues is most strongly related to slow gait speed (i.e., <0.8 m/s) and frailty [11]. Moreover, the Alcazar EQ predicts numerous physical health-related variables, such as usual gait speed (UGS) and fast gait speed (FGS), timed up-and-go (TUG) performance, health-related quality of life, hospitalizations, and mortality in aging populations [8,11,12]. Importantly, EQ STS power is sensitive to intervention [13,14], and its improvement is significantly associated with augmented PF [14]. Therefore, EQ STS power could be used as a clinically useful, valid, and sensitive method to monitor aging adults' muscle power.

While some research groups have developed EQs to estimate STS power, others have developed instrumented protocols using force plates [15,16], wearable monitors/accelerometers [17,18], and linear position transducers (LPTs) [5,19,20]. LPTs are relatively affordable, portable, and have the benefit of providing instantaneous, objective feedback to both patient and provider, with minimal data processing. Of clinical importance, LPT STS power is significantly associated with the Short Physical Performance Battery, gait speed, TUG performance, and balance in aging adults [20–22].

Multiple cut-off values for EQ STS power have recently been proposed and are associated with important aging outcomes such as sarcopenia, physical independence, mobility and frailty, ability to perform basic (BADL) and instrumental activities of daily living (IADL), hospitalizations, and poor quality of life [12,23–25]. For example, in a large sample of aging Spanish adults, EQ STS power cut-off values of 1.7 and 2.2 W/kg for females and males, respectively, have been proposed, and are associated with a greater likelihood of having poor PF (i.e., slow UGS, frailty, and limitations in ADLs and IADLs) [26]. Based on these proposed cut-off values, an operational clinical algorithm was developed to screen and manage the care of patients with low EQ STS power [26]. While not identifying cut-off values for low STS power, nor linking these data to PF outcomes, recently reported normative data in U.S. adults, using the TENDO LPT, report seemingly higher estimates of STS power [27] compared to the EQ STS power estimated in similar populations [23,25,26]. This suggests that STS power ascertained from different methods may yield considerably different estimates. Therefore, caution should be used when qualitatively describing patients' STS power to make clinical decisions.

Discrepancies of STS power estimates between methods could be due to differences in test procedures. Specifically, EQ STS power is estimated from five consecutive STS transitions [1], whereas LPT STS power is assessed from one maximal effort stand from a seated position [20,27]. For the future screening and management of low muscle power in the clinical setting, it is important to establish the agreement between different methods. Doing so will determine whether proposed cut-off values can be applied across methods, or if method-specific cut-off values are required. Moreover, evaluating whether STS power methods differ in their relationships with PF outcomes in aging adults is important from a method selection perspective. Importantly, some evidence suggests that EQ STS power may predict TUG performance better than more objective, technology-based assessments [15,28,29]. However, to the authors' knowledge, no study has directly compared the strengths of the relationships between different STS power methods and multiple objective and self-reported PF outcomes. Therefore, limited conclusions can be made regarding the relative ability of these methods to predict PF in aging adults.

The aims of this study, therefore, were to assess the absolute agreement between EQ and LPT STS power and to compare the relationships between EQ and LPT STS power assessments with objective and self-reported PF in aging adults. Based on previous estimates [26,27], we hypothesized that EQ and LPT STS power will showcase limited absolute agreement, with LPT STS power demonstrating consistently higher estimates than EQ STS power. Furthermore, based on limited, indirect evidence [15,29], we hypothesized that EQ STS power may demonstrate stronger relationships with PF outcomes compared to LPT STS power. The results of this study may have important implications for the future screening and management of low muscle power in the clinical setting.

2. Materials and Methods

2.1. Participants

Participants were recruited for this cross-sectional study via print and digital flyers, posted throughout various neighborhoods and businesses near a large, midwestern, urban university in the United States, and online via social media posts. Participants were eligible to participate in the study if they (1) were 40+ years of age, (2) could stand from a chair once and walk 10 m without the assistance of another person, and (3) could speak and read English. Participants were excluded from the study if they (1) used a wheelchair for mobility purposes, (2) were unable to safely follow the study procedures, or (3) had a resting heart rate or blood pressure over 100 bpm or 160/100 mmHg, respectively. Participants did not receive any financial compensation for their participation in this study, and all study procedures were reviewed and approved by the University of Wisconsin-Milwaukee's institutional review board (protocol #23.133 on 6 January 2023). Participant recruitment and data collection for this study occurred between March 2023 and April 2024.

2.2. Sociodemographic Variables, Anthropometrics, and Body Composition

Sociodemographic and health history information were collected with a study-specific questionnaire. Participant body height and mass were measured with a calibrated stadiometer and physician's scale, respectively (Detecto, Webb City, MO, USA). Body mass index (BMI) was calculated as body mass to height, squared (kg/m^2).

2.3. STS Power Assessments

Randomization of the STS test order was performed by the lead author (G.S.) in February 2023, before beginning data collection. Both STS tests were completed on a 0.45 m-tall armless chair. For both assessments, participants began seated in the middle of the chair, with their feet flat on the floor and arms crossed over their chest, to limit the use of their upper extremities. To maintain ecological validity, no instruction was given with respect to starting ankle or knee joint angles [27].

To calculate EQ STS power, the total time for participants to perform 5 consecutive STS transitions, as quickly as possible, was measured to the nearest hundredths of a second with a manual stopwatch. The timing of the test began after the researcher said, "Ready, set, go!", and stopped when the participant was seated on the fifth repetition [15]. The following validated EQ was used to estimate relative mean STS power [1]:

$$Absolute\ STS\ mean\ power\ (\mathrm{W}) = \frac{Body\ mass \times 0.9 \times g \times [\mathrm{Body}\ height \times 0.5 - \mathrm{Chair}\ height]}{\mathrm{Five\ STS}\ time \times 0.1} \quad (1)$$

$$Relative\ STS\ mean\ power\ \left(\frac{\mathrm{W}}{\mathrm{kg}}\right) = \frac{Absolute\ STS\ mean\ power}{Body\ mass} \quad (2)$$

where body mass is entered in kilograms, g is the gravitational constant 9.81, body height and chair height are entered in meters, and the time to complete five STS transitions are entered as seconds.

The LPT STS test was conducted as described by Sherwood and colleagues [20]. Briefly, the GymAware LPT, a valid and reliable LPT to assess STS power in aging adults [20], was positioned on a metal plate situated 8 cm lateral and 36 cm anterior to the back leg of the armless chair, and the unit's tether was attached to the participant's hip via a gait belt. Due to the feet and shank regions not being displaced during the STS transition, 90% of the participant's body mass was entered into the GymAware iPad application (GymAware 3.2.3; Kinetic Performance Technology, Braddon, ACT, Australia) prior to the test. After the researcher explained the test protocol, participants were told to stand, as quickly as possible, from the chair a total of 5 separate times, with 1 min of rest given between each stand [20]. Mean and peak instantaneous velocity, force, and power parameters were estimated from each trial and later exported from the GymAware Cloud Pro software (https://gymaware.com/shop/#gymaware-cloud (accessed on 6 January 2023)). The maximal relative mean STS power elicited during the test was used for analysis.

2.4. Objective Physical Function Outcomes

Handgrip strength (HGS) is a proxy of overall muscle strength and is used to diagnose sarcopenia, or the age-related loss of skeletal muscle mass, strength, and function [30]. Participants sat on an adjustable chair, with their forearm resting on an adjustable table and their elbow joint flexed at approximately 90 degrees. The chair and table's heights were adjusted to ensure the participants' shoulders were level. After familiarization, participants were instructed to squeeze a calibrated hand dynamometer (Lafayette Professional Hand Dynamometer FE-12-5203, Lafayette Instrument, Lafayette, IN, USA) as hard as possible for five seconds. After each trial, participants were given 30 s of rest. Participants completed three trials in each hand, with the first set of trials being completed with the participants' dominant hand. The maximal HGS attained over the six total trials was normalized to the participants' body mass and used for analysis.

The TUG test is a functional mobility test and is an indicator of balance, gait speed, and ADL performance in the aging population [31]. Briefly, participants started the test seated in a standard armchair 0.46 m in seat height and 0.65 m in arm rest height. Participants were instructed to stand from the chair, walk around a cone situated 3 m away, return to the chair, and sit back down at their usual pace. The time taken to complete the test was measured on a stopwatch, measured to the nearest hundredths of a second.

The 10 m walk test is a valid and reliable assessment of gait speed in the adult population [32]. Gait speed is a potent predictor of mortality, mobility disability, and falls, and is often cited as the "functional vital sign" [33–36]. Given that UGS and FGS differ in their relationships to PF in community-dwelling aging adults [37], we assessed gait speed at both velocities. For the assessment of UGS, participants were instructed to walk 10 m down an unobstructed corridor at their usual, comfortable pace, while for the assessment of FGS, participants were instructed to walk the same distance at their maximal walking pace, without running. To account for acceleration and deceleration, the timed portion of the test included only the intermediate 6 m of the 10 m track. A researcher timed the participants with a manual stopwatch, to the nearest hundredths of a second, and UGS and FGS were estimated for each trial. Participants completed 3 trials of both UGS and FGS, and the average of the 3 trials was used for analysis.

The fast-paced 400 m walk test (400MWT) is a valid predictor of aerobic fitness in aging adults [38]. Each 1 min longer 400MWT time is associated with a ~30% increase in all-cause mortality [39], and the inability to complete the test is associated with a near two-fold greater risk of future mobility limitations and disability [40]. To complete the test, two cones were placed 20 m apart in an unobstructed corridor. Participants were instructed to complete 10 laps around the 40 m track, walking at their maximal pace, without running. Participants were allowed to stop twice throughout the test, if needed, but were told that the time would continue during rest periods. Time taken to complete the test was measured to the nearest second with a manual stopwatch.

2.5. Self-Report Physical Function

The Late-Life Function and Disability Instrument (LLFDI) is a valid self-report measure of PF in aging adults, with moderately strong relationships demonstrated between LLFDI subscales and objective assessments of function (i.e., SPPB and 400MWT performance) [41]. For this study, the functional domain of the LLFDI contains the primary outcomes of interest. Specifically, the scaled scores (0–100) of total, basic lower-body, and advanced lower-body function were the outcomes.

2.6. Power Calculation

A post hoc power calculation was performed in the pwr R package (v1.3.0). Assuming a mean difference and pooled standard deviation between EQ and LPT STS power estimates of 1.5 and 1.15 W/kg, respectively [23,27], 50 participants result in a power = 1.0, and, therefore, a 100% probability of detecting a mean difference of this magnitude or greater between methods.

2.7. Statistical Analysis

Continuous and categorical descriptive statistics are reported as mean (SD) and *n* (%), respectively. The absolute agreement between STS power methods was assessed by calculating an intraclass correlation coefficient (ICC) using the icc R package (v2.4.0) and constructing a Bland–Altman plot [42] using the blandr (v0.6.0) and ggplot2 (v3.5.2) R packages. The ICC and Bland–Altman methods are recommended to evaluate the agreement between continuous variables [43]. The unadjusted and adjusted relationships between STS power assessments and PF outcomes were assessed with Pearson product–moment correlation coefficients and multiple linear regression, respectively. Based on previous research [15], age, as a continuous variable, and sex, as a dichotomous variable, were selected as covariates a priori in the multiple linear regression models. Using the gtsummary R package (v2.1.0), standardized beta coefficients and their 95% confidence intervals are reported to compare the strengths of the associations between STS power methods and PF outcomes. All statistical analyses were completed in R (v4.4.2), using an alpha level of 0.05 for statistical significance.

3. Results

Overall, 94 participants were screened for eligibility, 50 participants completed all study procedures, and, due to data retrieval issues with the GymAware, 49 participants were included in the final analytic sample (Figure 1). A summary of participant characteristics is shown in Table 1.

Mean EQ and LPT STS power were 2.95 (0.98) and 5.69 (1.64) W/kg, respectively, with moderate agreement demonstrated between methods (ICC3 = 0.69 [0.51, 0.81]). The Bland–Altman plot is shown in Figure 2. Mean bias [95%CI] between EQ and LPT power was 2.73 W/kg [95%CI: 2.43, 3.04]. Additionally, there was a moderately strong positive relationship between average STS power performance and bias between methods ($r = 0.66$).

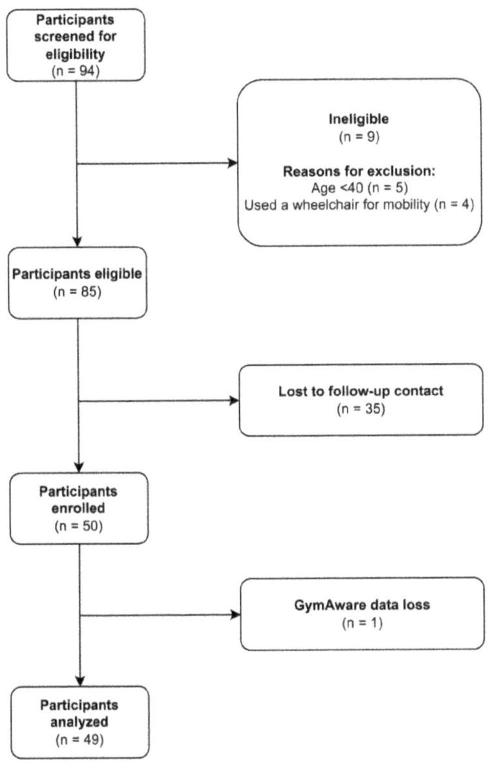

Figure 1. Participant inclusion/exclusion flowchart.

Table 1. Participant characteristics.

Characteristic	N = 49 [1]
Age, years	61 (11)
Sex	
Male	16 (33%)
Female	33 (67%)
Race and ethnicity	
Hispanic	1 (2.0%)
NH Asian	1 (2.0%)
NH Black	1 (2.0%)
NH White	44 (90%)
NH More than one race	2 (4.1%)
BMI, kg/m^2	26.4 (5.2)
EQ STS power, W/kg	2.95 (0.98)
LPT STS power, W/kg	5.69 (1.64)
Handgrip strength, kg/kg	0.47 (0.13)
Timed up-and-go, s	8.98 (1.81)
Usual gait speed, m/s	1.37 (0.20)
Fast gait speed, m/s	2.01 (0.34)
400 m walk, s	248 (44)
LLFDI total physical function	81 (12)
LLFDI basic lower-body physical function	92 (11)
LLFDI advanced lower-body physical function	79 (15)

[1] Mean (SD) and n (%) for continuous and categorical variables, respectively; NH = non-Hispanic, BMI = body mass index, EQ = equation, STS = sit-to-stand, LPT = linear position transducer, LLFDI = Late-Life Function and Disability Instrument.

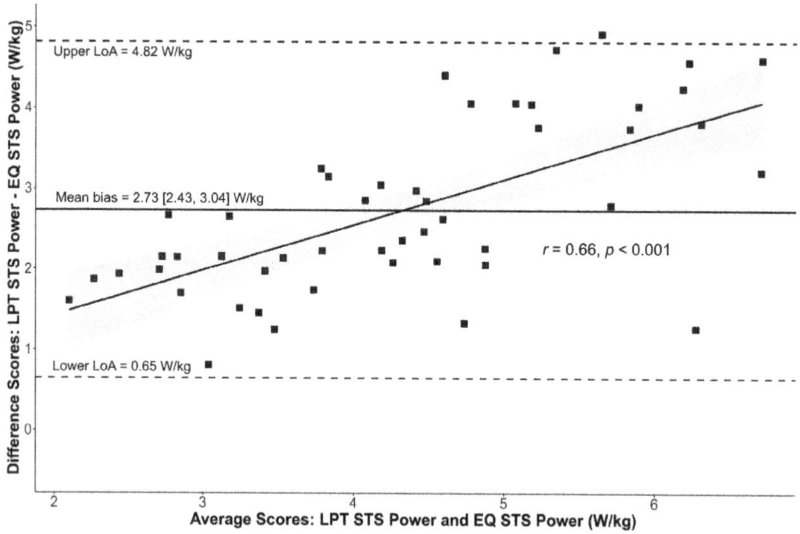

Figure 2. Bland–Altman plot, illustrating the mean bias and limits of agreement (LoA) between EQ and LPT STS power.

The unadjusted relationships between STS power methods are shown in Table 2. Overall, both EQ and LPT STS power were significantly associated with all PF outcomes ($p < 0.01$). Aside from HGS, EQ STS power showcased similar or marginally stronger associations with PF outcomes as LPT STS power.

Table 2. Unadjusted relationships (r) between EQ and LPT STS power and physical function outcomes.

Variable	Handgrip Strength	Timed Up-and-Go	Usual Gait Speed	Fast Gait Speed	400 m Walk Test	LLFDI Total Function	LLFDI Basic Lower-Body Function	LLFDI Advanced Lower-Body Function
EQ STS power	**0.37**	**−0.52**	**0.49**	**0.61**	**−0.70**	**0.54**	**0.51**	**0.51**
LPT STS power	**0.53**	**−0.38**	**0.42**	**0.55**	**−0.67**	**0.52**	**0.48**	**0.51**

EQ = equation, LPT = linear position transducer, STS = sit-to-stand, LLFDI = Late-Life Function and Disability Instrument. Bolded correlation coefficients are statistically significant at $\alpha = 0.05$.

The multivariate regression analyses examining the independent associations between STS power methods and objective PF outcomes are shown in Table 3. Controlling for age and sex, EQ STS power was associated with TUG (Std. $\beta = -0.45$ [95%CI: −0.74, −0.17]), UGS (Std. $\beta = 0.37$ [95%CI: 0.08, 0.66]), FGS (Std. $\beta = 0.48$ [95%CI: 0.23, 0.74]), and 400MWT (Std. $\beta = -0.55$ [95%CI: −0.77, −0.33]), but not HGS (Std. $\beta = 0.19$ [95%CI: −0.10, 0.48]). Controlled for the same confounders, LPT STS power was significantly associated with HGS (Std. $\beta = 0.44$ [95%CI: 0.18, 0.70]), FGS (Std. $\beta = 0.40$ [95%CI: 0.14, 0.66]) and 400MWT (Std. $\beta = -0.51$ [95%CI: −0.73, −0.29]), but neither TUG (Std. $\beta = -0.26$ [95%CI: −0.56, 0.04]) nor UGS (Std. $\beta = 0.28$ [−0.01, 0.57]).

Table 3. Adjusted relationships between EQ and LPT STS power and objective physical function outcomes.

	Handgrip Strength		Timed Up-and-Go		Usual Gait Speed		Fast Gait Speed		400 m Walk Test	
	Std. β	95% CI	Std. β	95% CI	Std. β	95% CI	Std. β	95% CI	Std. β	95% CI
EQ STS power	0.19	−0.10, 0.48	**−0.45**	**−0.74, −0.17**	**0.37**	**0.08, 0.66**	**0.48**	**0.23, 0.74**	**−0.55**	**−0.77, −0.33**
LPT STS power	**0.44**	**0.18, 0.70**	−0.26	−0.56, 0.04	0.28	−0.01, 0.57	**0.40**	**0.14, 0.66**	**−0.51**	**−0.73, −0.29**

Std. = standardized, CI = confidence interval, EQ = equation, STS = sit-to-stand, LPT = linear position transducer. Bolded Std. β and 95% CI are statistically significant at α = 0.05. All models are adjusted for age (continuous) + sex (dichotomous).

The multivariate regression analyses examining the associations between STS power methods and self-reported PF are shown in Table 4. Both EQ and LPT STS power were statistically and similarly associated with self-reported total (Std. βs = 0.30–0.31), basic lower-body (Std. βs = 0.29–0.30), and advanced lower-body function (Std. βs = 0.30–0.32), independent of age and sex.

Table 4. Adjusted relationships between EQ and LPT STS power and self-reported physical function outcomes.

	LLFDI Total Function		LLFDI Basic Lower-Body Function		LLFDI Advanced Lower-Body Function	
	Std. β	95% CI	Std. β	95% CI	Std. β	95% CI
EQ STS power	**0.30**	**0.05, 0.55**	**0.30**	**0.04, 0.57**	**0.30**	**0.03, 0.57**
LPT STS power	**0.31**	**0.07, 0.55**	**0.29**	**0.03, 0.55**	**0.32**	**0.06, 0.58**

Std. = standardized, CI = confidence interval, EQ = equation, STS = sit-to-stand, LPT = linear position transducer, LLFDI = Late-Life Function and Disability Instrument. Bolded Std. β and 95% CI are statistically significant at α = 0.05. All models are adjusted for age (continuous) + sex (dichotomous).

4. Discussion

The purpose of this study was to evaluate the agreement between EQ and LPT STS power in a sample of aging adults. Additionally, this study compared the strengths of the associations between STS power methods and PF outcomes. In line with our hypothesis, EQ and LPT STS power demonstrated limited agreement, suggesting that proposed cut-off values to identify low muscle power [23,26] should not be applied across different methodologies. Interestingly, EQ STS power seems to be similarly or more strongly associated with PF outcomes compared to LPT STS power, suggesting EQ STS power may act as a superior proxy for PF in aging adults. Given that the EQ STS power test requires relatively less time and financial resources, and less test administration expertise, its feasibility for use as a screening tool in the clinical setting should be explored further.

The finding that EQ and LPT STS power demonstrate limited agreement is clinically important, as multiple cut-off values to detect low muscle power have been proposed [23,26]. Additionally, while no clinically meaningful change in STS power has been identified [29], some research groups have proposed STS power thresholds to identify mobility limitations and disability [26,44]. Therefore, evaluating the agreement between STS power estimates of different methods is paramount for muscle power screening in clinical settings. Screening for and ameliorating low muscle power is likely to improve PF [4,14], reduce falls [16], and may promote longevity in aging adults [8,12]. The limited agreement between EQ and LPT STS power reported in this study is consistent with published normative data [23,25,27]. Indeed, Campitelli and colleagues recently reported normative STS power across the lifespan using a TENDO LPT [27]. In this study, average relative mean STS power, which was assessed in adults aged 50–80, ranged from 4 to 7.5 W/kg, which is notably higher than published EQ STS power estimates in large cohorts of similarly aged Spanish and

Colombian adults [23,25], but similar to the results of this study. Given that an algorithm has been developed to detect and manage low STS power in the clinical setting [26], if multiple methods are to be used to assess STS power, method-specific cut-off values should be developed and validated in functionally and clinically diverse populations. Moreover, the feasibility of implementing STS power tests and their associated cut-off values into diverse clinical settings should be explored.

Reasons why STS power estimates differ quite drastically between methods are likely due to differences in test procedures. Specifically, EQ STS power estimates the velocity, and therefore power, of one concentric phase of the STS transition from five repeated transitions, assuming that the durations of the concentric and eccentric phases of these transitions are identical. It is likely, however, especially in aging adults, that the duration of each subsequent STS transition in a multiple-transition test (i.e., five-repetition STS test) increases over the test duration, due to the accumulation of fatigue. This, therefore, would result in an underestimation of STS velocity, which has been demonstrated previously [45]. On the other hand, LPTs precisely measure velocity [46], and therefore power, of a single concentric phase of the STS transition. Given that we assumed the same input of force (i.e., 90% of the participant's body weight) for both tests, an underestimation of velocity will necessarily result in lower STS power values, which are clearly illustrated in this study.

Interestingly, however, EQ STS power was similarly, and in many cases, more strongly associated with PF outcomes compared to LPT STS power. It is perhaps unsurprising that EQ STS power was a stronger predictor of PF outcomes, as longer-duration STS tests are consistently more strongly associated with 6 min walk performance in both young, apparently healthy adults [47], and in adults with chronic obstructive pulmonary disease [48]. Moreover, performance in the 30 and 60 s variations of the STS test better predict performance in HGS, cognitive tasks, quality of life, and fatigue in older adults, compared to shorter-duration STS tests, such as the five-repetition STS test [49]. While this is the first study to directly compare the relationships between EQ and LPT STS power and PF outcomes in aging adults, the current study's findings generally comport with the existing literature. Specifically, Baltasar-Fernandez and colleagues assessed the relationship between EQ STS power and PF outcomes [15], while Balachandran et al. have investigated the relationships between LPT STS power and PF outcomes using both the TENDO and GymAware LPTs [21,29]. In these studies, the unadjusted relationships between STS power and TUG performance, for example, were stronger when using EQ STS power ($r = 0.59$), compared to LPT STS power ($r = 0.41$–0.53), as the primary independent variable. However, these previous studies are limited by not measuring EQ and LPT STS power concurrently. In comparing these previous findings with the results of this study, therefore, EQ STS power and LPT STS power demonstrated unadjusted relationships with TUG performances of $r = 0.52$ and 0.38, respectively. Importantly, these differences in the relationships between STS power methods and PF outcomes persisted when adjusted for confounding variables (i.e., age and sex) and across most objective PF outcomes. Based on the results of this study, it appears that EQ STS power provides similar if not greater clarity into aging adults' PF compared to LPT STS power, and its preferential use in the clinical setting may be justified as a result.

These findings suggesting EQ STS power, ascertained from the five-repetition STS test, is a better indicator of aging adults' PF compared to LPT STS power may be due to a relatively large "reserve" of maximal lower-body muscle strength [50], and consequently, muscle power, when performing PF-related tasks in this population. It could, therefore, be the case that the ability to sustain muscular force and power over relatively longer periods of time (i.e., muscular endurance) is more important for from a functional perspective compared to producing maximal force and power, which is partially confirmed by the results of this current study. Indeed, while LPT STS power was more strongly associated with maximal strength (i.e., HGS) compared to EQ STS power, it was more weakly associated with ambulatory PF outcomes, which are stronger predictors of mobility limitations, falls, and mortality [51]. Additionally, PF and frailty indicators are improved to a similar degree in adults 65+ years of age randomized to resistance training (RT) or aerobic training, despite preferential increases in maximal strength after RT [52]. This suggests that maximal force production is generally not the limiting factor in maintaining PF into late adulthood and perhaps explains why LPT STS power demonstrated weaker relationships with PF outcomes compared to EQ STS power. Given that EQ STS power is validated to quantify power during both the 5 [1] and 30 s iterations of the STS test [53], and normative data have been published for both [23,25,44], future research should examine whether EQ STS power estimates agree across different test variations, and also determine if they similarly predict PF outcomes in aging adults. The results of this future investigation could better inform the selection of the most functionally relevant STS test to screen for muscle power in the clinical setting.

One limitation of this study is its relatively young and high-functioning sample of aging adults. Therefore, it is unclear whether our findings would be replicated in a sample of older and/or physically lower-functioning adults. Specific to our agreement analyses, we identified a moderately strong linear relationship (r = 0.66) between STS power performance and the bias between STS power methods, whereby higher average STS power was associated with greater bias. Therefore, it could be the case that these two methods agree when examining the STS power of adults with relatively low muscle power. However, given the large bias demonstrated in the current study, in addition to observable differences in normative STS power values between methods across the aging spectrum [25–27], it is unlikely that high levels of agreement would be demonstrated, even at extremely low levels of muscle power. Future research may aim to investigate this further, however. With respect to comparing the associations between STS power methods and PF outcomes, it is reasonable that, in an older and/or physically lower-functioning sample, with relatively less strength and power reserve, maximal power could be relatively more important for PF, perhaps resulting in similar or stronger associations between LPT STS power and PF outcomes, compared to EQ STS power. While this could be the case, longer-duration STS tests are consistently more strongly related to PF outcomes in aging adults compared to shorter-duration STS tests [48,49]. Relatedly, it is unclear whether the observed differences in the relationships between STS power estimates and PF are clinically meaningful. For example, in this study, a 1-SD greater EQ and LPT STS power was associated with a 0.37 and 0.28-SD greater UGS, which corresponds to 0.07 and 0.06 m/s, respectively. Given that the clinically meaningful difference in UGS has been cited as 0.05–0.12 m/s [54], these differences may be negligible. Nonetheless, the main questions of this study should be examined in a larger and more functionally diverse sample. Similarly, 90% of the participants in this study were non-Hispanic White, which limits its external validity. Studies with greater demographic variability should be conducted to test the generalizability of our findings. Larger studies should also be conducted to examine the moderating roles of age and sex on the relationships between STS power estimates and PF outcomes, and to determine whether method-specific cut-off values differ between patient populations. Finally, while EQ STS power shows stronger cross-sectional associations with PF outcomes compared to LPT STS power, it is unclear whether EQ STS power would be a superior predictor of "harder" clinical endpoints (e.g., mobility disability, falls, mortality). Future research should investigate the prospective associations between different STS power variations and these important clinical outcomes.

One notable strength of this study is its direct comparison between two common methods of assessing STS power in aging adults. As such, the findings from this study are pragmatic, and may inform the future implementation of screening for muscle power in the clinical setting. Another strength of this study is its use of not only objective PF outcomes but also self-reported PF outcomes, which are increasingly recognized as valuable patient data, as they provide unique information regarding a patient's condition and abilities not otherwise captured by more objective PF outcomes [55].

5. Conclusions

This study compared the agreement between two STS power methods, in addition to evaluating the strengths of the associations between these methods and PF outcomes. Overall, STS power, estimated from the five-repetition STS test and from an LPT, demonstrate limited agreement. Therefore, the estimates from different STS power methods should not be used interchangeably, and the use of current and future cut-off values for low STS power should be specific to the method used. STS power, ascertained from the five-repetition STS test, is, in general, more strongly related with objective PF outcomes compared to LPT STS power. However, future research should elucidate the clinical implications of this and investigate whether EQ STS power better predicts "harder" clinical endpoints (e.g., mobility disability, falls, mortality) compared to LPT STS power. After replicating these findings in a larger, more demographically and clinically heterogeneous sample, future work should assess the feasibility of implementing STS power assessments as screening tools in the clinical setting. Identifying and referring patients with low muscle power to effective therapeutic interventions to improve muscle power (e.g., exercise interventions) [14] may prevent and ameliorate the negative individual and population health consequences of low muscle power.

Author Contributions: Conceptualization, G.S., T.D. and S.S.; methodology, G.S., T.D. and S.S.; formal analysis, G.S.; investigation, G.S., T.D., J.M. and J.P.; resources, A.S. and S.S.; writing—original draft preparation, G.S.; writing—review and editing, T.D., J.M., J.P., A.S. and S.S.; visualization, G.S. and J.M.; supervision, S.S.; project administration, G.S. All authors have read and agreed to the published version of the manuscript.

Funding: This research received no external funding.

Institutional Review Board Statement: This study was conducted in accordance with the Declaration of Helsinki and approved by the Institutional Review Board of the University of Wisconsin-Milwaukee (protocol #23.133; approved on 6 January 2023).

Informed Consent Statement: Informed consent was obtained from all subjects involved in the study.

Data Availability Statement: The raw data supporting the conclusions of this article will be made available by the authors on request.

Acknowledgments: The authors would like to sincerely thank the participants who participated in this study. The authors would also like to sincerely thank Cloe Belongia and Katharine O'Connell-Valuch for their invaluable administrative support.

Conflicts of Interest: The authors declare no conflicts of interest.

Abbreviations

The following abbreviations are used in this manuscript:

PF	physical function
EQ	equation
STS	sit-to-stand
UGS	usual gait speed

FGS	fast gait speed
TUG	timed up-and-go
LPT	linear position transducer
BMI	body mass index
HGS	handgrip strength
400MWT	400 m walk test
LLFDI	Late-Life Function and Disability Instrument
Std. β	standardized beta coefficient

References

1. Alcazar, J.; Losa-Reyna, J.; Rodriguez-Lopez, C.; Alfaro-Acha, A.; Rodriguez-Mañas, L.; Ara, I.; García-García, F.J.; Alegre, L.M. The sit-to-stand muscle power test: An easy, inexpensive and portable procedure to assess muscle power in older people. *Exp. Gerontol.* **2018**, *112*, 38–43. [CrossRef] [PubMed]
2. Reid, K.F.; Fielding, R.A. Skeletal Muscle Power: A Critical Determinant of Physical Functioning in Older Adults. *Exerc. Sport Sci. Rev.* **2012**, *40*, 4–12. [CrossRef]
3. Bean, J.F.; Kiely, D.K.; Herman, S.; Leveille, S.G.; Mizer, K.; Frontera, W.R.; Fielding, R.A. The Relationship Between Leg Power and Physical Performance in Mobility-Limited Older People. *J. Am. Geriatr. Soc.* **2002**, *50*, 461–467. [PubMed]
4. Bean, J.F.; Kiely, D.K.; Larose, S.; Goldstein, R.; Frontera, W.R.; Leveille, S.G. Are changes in leg power responsible for clinically meaningful improvements in mobility in older adults? *J. Am. Geriatr. Soc.* **2010**, *58*, 2363–2368. [CrossRef]
5. Orange, S.T.; Metcalfe, J.W.; Liefeith, A.; Jordan, A.R. Validity of various portable devices to measure sit-to-stand velocity and power in older adults. *Gait Posture* **2020**, *76*, 409–414. [CrossRef]
6. Simpkins, C.; Yang, F. Muscle power is more important than strength in preventing falls in community-dwelling older adults. *J. Biomech.* **2022**, *134*, 111018. [CrossRef]
7. Steinbrink, G.M.; Martinez, J.; Swartz, A.M.; Strath, S.J. Sit-to-Stand Power Is a Stronger Predictor of Gait Speed than Knee Extension Strength. *J. Funct. Morphol. Kinesiol.* **2024**, *9*, 103. [CrossRef]
8. Alcazar, J.; Navarrete-, D.; Mañas, A.; Alegre, L.M.; Villa, G.; Cabello, A.G.-; Pedrero-, R.; Gusi, N.; González-, M.; Casajús, J.A.; et al. 'Fat but powerful ' paradox: Association of muscle power and adiposity markers with all-cause mortality in older adults from the EXERNET multicentre study. *Br. J. Sports Med.* **2021**, *55*, 1204–1211. [CrossRef]
9. Freitas, S.; Cruz-Montecinos, C.; Ratel, S.; Pinto, R. Powerpenia: Should it be considered a biomarker of healthy aging? *Sports Med.-Open* **2024**, *10*, 27. [CrossRef]
10. Alcazar, J.; Guadalupe-Grau, A.; García-García, F.J.; Ara, I.; Alegre, L.M. Skeletal Muscle Power Measurement in Older People: A Systematic Review of Testing Protocols and Adverse Events. *J. Gerontol.-Ser. A Biol. Sci. Med. Sci.* **2018**, *73*, 914–924. [CrossRef]
11. Baltasar-Fernandez, I.; Alcazar, J.; Losa-Reyna, J.; Soto-Paniagua, H.; Alegre, L.M.; Takai, Y.; Ruiz-Cárdenas, J.D.; Signorile, J.F.; Rodriguez-Mañas, L.; García-García, F.J.; et al. Comparison of available equations to estimate sit-to-stand muscle power and their association with gait speed and frailty in older people: Practical applications for the 5-rep sit-to-stand test. *Exp. Gerontol.* **2021**, *156*, 111619. [CrossRef] [PubMed]
12. Losa-Reyna, J.; Alcazar, J.; Carnicero, J.; Alfaro-Acha, A.; Castillo-Gallego, C.; Rosado-Artalejo, C.; Rodríguez-Mañas, L.; Ara, I.; García-García, F.J. Impact of Relative Muscle Power on Hospitalization and All-Cause Mortality in Older Adults. *J. Gerontol. Ser. A* **2021**, *77*, 781–789. [CrossRef] [PubMed]
13. Baltasar-Fernandez, I.; Alcazar, J.; Martín-Braojos, S.; Ara, I.; Alegre, L.M.; García-García, F.J.; Alfaro-Acha, A.; Losa-Reyna, J. Power-oriented resistance training combined with high-intensity interval training in pre-frail and frail older people: Comparison between traditional and cluster training set configurations on the force–velocity relationship, physical function and frailty. *Eur. J. Appl. Physiol.* **2023**, *124*, 623–632. [CrossRef]
14. Lanzi, S.; Pousaz, A.; Calanca, L.; Mazzolai, L. Sit-to-stand muscle power is related to functional performance at baseline and after supervised exercise training in patients with lower extremity peripheral artery disease. *Eur. J. Vasc. Endovasc. Surg.* **2022**, *65*, 512–527. [CrossRef]
15. Baltasar-Fernandez, I.; Alcazar, J.; Rodriguez-Lopez, C.; Losa-Reyna, J.; Alonso-Seco, M.; Ara, I.; Alegre, L.M. Sit-to-stand muscle power test: Comparison between estimated and force plate-derived mechanical power and their association with physical function in older adults. *Exp. Gerontol.* **2021**, *145*, 111213. [CrossRef] [PubMed]
16. Cheng, Y.Y.; Wei, S.H.; Chen, P.Y.; Tsai, M.W.; Cheng, I.C.; Liu, D.H.; Kao, C.L. Can sit-to-stand lower limb muscle power predict fall status? *Gait Posture* **2014**, *40*, 403–407. [CrossRef]
17. Tateoka, K.; Tsuji, T.; Shoji, T.; Tokunaga, S.; Okura, T. Relationship between Acceleration in a Sit-To-Stand Movement and Physical Function in Older Adults. *Geriatrics* **2023**, *8*, 123. [CrossRef]

18. Van Lummel, R.C.; Walgaard, S.; Maier, A.B.; Ainsworth, E.; Beek, P.J.; Van Dieën, J.H. The instrumented Sit-To-Stand test (iSTS) has greater clinical relevance than the manually recorded sit-to-stand test in older adults. *PLoS ONE* **2016**, *11*, e0157968. [CrossRef]
19. Gray, M.; Paulson, S. Developing a measure of muscular power during a functional task for older adults. *BMC Geriatr.* **2014**, *14*, 145. [CrossRef]
20. Sherwood, J.J.; Inouye, C.; Webb, S.L.; Jenny, O. Reliability and validity of the sit-to-stand as a muscular power measure in older adults. *J. Aging Phys. Act.* **2020**, *28*, 455–466. [CrossRef]
21. Balachandran, A.T.; Vigotsky, A.D.; Quiles, N.; Mokkink, L.B.; Belio, M.A.; Glenn, J.M.K. Validity, reliability, and measurement error of a sit-to-stand power test in older adults: A pre-registered study. *Exp. Gerontol.* **2021**, *145*, 111202. [CrossRef] [PubMed]
22. Glenn, J.M.; Gray, M.; Binns, A. Relationship of Sit-to-Stand Lower-Body Power With Functional Fitness Measures Among Older Adults With and Without Sarcopenia. *J. Geriatr. Phys. Ther.* **2017**, *40*, 42–50. [CrossRef] [PubMed]
23. Alcazar, J.; Alegre, L.M.; Van Roie, E.; Magalhães, J.P.; Nielsen, B.R.; González-Gross, M.; Júdice, P.B.; Casajús, J.A.; Delecluse, C.; Sardinha, L.B.; et al. Relative sit-to-stand power: Aging trajectories, functionally relevant cut-off points, and normative data in a large European cohort. *J. Cachexia Sarcopenia Muscle* **2021**, *12*, 921–932. [CrossRef]
24. Hetherington-Rauth, M.; Magalhães, J.P.; Alcazar, J.; Rosa, G.B.; Correia, I.R.; Ara, I.; Sardinha, L.B. Relative Sit-to-Stand Muscle Power Predicts an Older Adult's Physical Independence at Age of 90 Yrs Beyond That of Relative Handgrip Strength, Physical Activity, and Sedentary Time: A Cross-sectional Analysis. *Am. J. Phys. Med. Rehabil.* **2022**, *101*, 995–1000. [CrossRef]
25. Ramírez-Vélez, R.; Izquierdo, M.; García-Hermoso, A.; Ordoñez-Mora, L.T.; Cano-Gutierrez, C.; Campo-Lucumí, F.; Pérez-Sousa, M.Á. Sit to stand muscle power reference values and their association with adverse events in Colombian older adults. *Sci. Rep.* **2022**, *12*, 11820. [CrossRef]
26. Losa-Reyna, J.; Alcazar, J.; Rodríguez-Gómez, I.; Alfaro-Acha, A.; Alegre, L.M.; Rodríguez-Mañas, L.; Ara, I.; García-García, F.J. Low relative mechanical power in older adults: An operational definition and algorithm for its application in the clinical setting. *Exp. Gerontol.* **2020**, *142*, 111141. [CrossRef] [PubMed]
27. Campitelli, A.; Paulson, S.; Vincenzo, J.; Glenn, J.M.; Gills, J.L.; Jones, M.D.; Powers, M.; Gray, M. Sit-to-Stand Power Across the Lifespan: A Cross-Sectional Analysis. *J. Aging Phys. Act.* **2021**, *30*, 678–688. [CrossRef]
28. Orange, S.T.; Marshall, P.; Madden, L.A.; Vince, R.V. Can sit-to-stand muscle power explain the ability to perform functional tasks in adults with severe obesity? *J. Sports Sci.* **2019**, *37*, 1227–1234. [CrossRef]
29. Balachandran, A.T.; Orange, S.T.; Wang, Y.; Lustin, R.; Vega, A.; Quiles, N. Comparison of two popular transducers to measure sit-to-stand power in older adults. *PLoS ONE* **2024**, *19*, e0308808. [CrossRef]
30. Vaishya, R.; Misra, A.; Vaish, A.; Ursino, N.; D'Ambrosi, R. Hand grip strength as a proposed new vital sign of health: A narrative review of evidences. *J. Health Popul. Nutr.* **2024**, *43*, 7. [CrossRef]
31. Podsiadlo, D.; Richardson, S. The Timed Up and Go: A Test of Basic Functional Mobility for Frail Elderly Persons. *J. Am. Geriatr. Soc.* **1991**, *39*, 142–148. [CrossRef] [PubMed]
32. Peters, D.M.; Fritz, S.L.; Krotish, D.E. Assessing the Reliability and Validity of a Shorter Walk Test Compared With the 10-Meter Walk Test for Measurements of Gait Speed in Healthy, Older Adults. *J. Geriatr. Phys. Ther.* **2013**, *36*, 24–30. [CrossRef]
33. Abellan Van Kan, G.; Rolland, Y.; Andrieu, S.; Bauer, J.; Beauchet, O.; Bonnefoy, M.; Cesari, M.; Donini, L.M.; Gillette-Guyonnet, S.; Inzitari, M.; et al. Gait speed at usual pace as a predictor of adverse outcomes in community-dwelling older people an International Academy on Nutrition and Aging (IANA) Task Force. *J. Nutr. Health Aging* **2009**, *13*, 881–889. [CrossRef] [PubMed]
34. McGrath, B.M.; Johnson, P.J.; Mcgrath, R.; Cawthon, P.M.; Klawitter, L.; Choi, B. A Matched Cohort Analysis for Examining the Association Between Slow Gait Speed and Shortened Longevity in Older Americans. *J. Appl. Gerontol.* **2022**, *41*, 1905–1913. [CrossRef] [PubMed]
35. Middleton, A.; Fritz, S.L.; Lusardi, M. Walking speed: The functional vital sign. *J. Aging Phys. Act.* **2015**, *23*, 314–322. [CrossRef]
36. Raisi, A.; Zerbini, V.; Myers, J.; Masotti, S.; Piva, T.; Lordi, R.; Chiaranda, G.; Grazzi, G.; Mazzoni, G.; Mandini, S. Moderate walking speed and survival association across 23-years follow-up in female patients with cardiovascular disease. *Int. J. Cardiol.* **2022**, *371*, 371–376. [CrossRef]
37. Gray, M.; Paulson, S.; Powers, M. Maximal, Not Habitual, Walking Velocity is More Highly Correlated to Functional Fitness of Community-Dwelling Older Adults. *J. Aging Phys. Act.* **2016**, *24*, 305–310. [CrossRef]
38. Simonsick, E.M.; Fan, E.; Fleg, J.L. Estimating Cardiorespiratory Fitness in Well-Functioning Older Adults: Treadmill Validation of the Long Distance Corridor Walk: Estimating Fitness in Older Adults. *J. Am. Geriatr. Soc.* **2006**, *54*, 127–132. [CrossRef]
39. Vestergaard, S.; Patel, K.V.; Bandinelli, S.; Ferrucci, L.; Guralnik, J.M. Characteristics of 400-meter walk test performance and subsequent mortality in older adults. *Rejuvenation Res.* **2009**, *12*, 177–184. [CrossRef]
40. Newman, A.B.; Simonsick, E.M.; Naydeck, B.L.; Boudreau, R.M.; Kritchevsky, S.B.; Nevitt, M.C.; Pahor, M.; Satterfield, S.; Brach, J.S.; Studenski, S.A.; et al. Association of Long-Distance Corridor Walk Performance With Mortality, Cardiovascular Disease, Mobility Limitation, and Disability. *JAMA* **2006**, *295*, 2018. [CrossRef]

41. Sayers, S.P.; Jette, A.M.; Haley, S.M.; Heeren, T.C.; Guralnik, J.M.; Fielding, R.A. Validation of the Late-Life Function and Disability Instrument: Validation of LLFDI. *J. Am. Geriatr. Soc.* **2004**, *52*, 1554–1559. [CrossRef] [PubMed]
42. Bland, J.M.; Altman, D.G. Statistical methods for assessing agreement between two methods of clinical measurement. *Int. J. Nurs. Stud.* **2010**, *47*, 931–936. [CrossRef]
43. Ranganathan, P.; Pramesh, C.; Aggarwal, R. Common pitfalls in statistical analysis: Measures of agreement. *Perspect. Clin. Res.* **2017**, *8*, 187. [CrossRef]
44. Garcia-Aguirre, M.; Baltasar-Fernandez, I.; Alcazar, J.; Losa-Reyna, J.; Alfaro-Acha, A.; Ara, I.; Rodriguez-Mañas, L.; Alegre, L.M.; Garcia-Garcia, F.J. Cut-Off Points for Low Relative 30-s Sit-to-Stand Power and Their Associations With Adverse Health Conditions. *J. Cachexia Sarcopenia Muscle* **2025**, *16*, e13676. [CrossRef] [PubMed]
45. Ferrari, L.; Bochicchio, G.; Bottari, A.; Lucertini, F.; Scarton, A.; Pogliaghi, S. Estimating Muscle Power of the Lower Limbs through the 5-Sit-to-Stand Test: A Comparison of Field vs. Laboratory Method. *Appl. Sci.* **2022**, *12*, 11577. [CrossRef]
46. Moreno-Villanueva, A.; Pino-Ortega, J.; Rico-González, M. Validity and reliability of linear position transducers and linear velocity transducers: A systematic review. *Sports Biomech.* **2021**, *23*, 1340–1369. [CrossRef]
47. Gurses, H.N.; Zeren, M.; Denizoglu Kulli, H.; Durgut, E. The relationship of sit-to-stand tests with 6-minute walk test in healthy young adults. *Medicine* **2018**, *97*, e9489. [CrossRef]
48. Gephine, S.; Frykholm, E.; Nyberg, A.; Mucci, P.; Van Hees, H.W.H.; Lemson, A.; Klijn, P.; Maltais, F.; Saey, D. Specific Contribution of Quadriceps Muscle Strength, Endurance, and Power to Functional Exercise Capacity in People With Chronic Obstructive Pulmonary Disease: A Multicenter Study. *Phys. Ther.* **2021**, *101*, pzab052. [CrossRef]
49. Stavrinou, P.S.; Aphamis, G.; Pantzaris, M.; Sakkas, G.K.; Giannaki, C.D. Exploring the Associations between Functional Capacity, Cognitive Function and Well-Being in Older Adults. *Life* **2022**, *12*, 1042. [CrossRef]
50. Hafer, J.F.; Boyer, K.A. Comparisons of knee extensor functional demand during gait by age, physical activity level, and the impact of acute exercise and walking speed. *J. Appl. Biomech.* **2020**, *36*, 163–170. [CrossRef]
51. Zanker, J.; Scott, D.; Alajlouni, D.; Kirk, B.; Bird, S.; DeBruin, D.; Vogrin, S.; Bliuc, D.; Tran, T.; Cawthon, P.; et al. Mortality, falls and slow walking speed are predicted by different muscle strength and physical performance measures in women and men. *Arch. Gerontol. Geriatr.* **2023**, *114*, 105084. [CrossRef] [PubMed]
52. Villareal, D.T.; Aguirre, L.; Gurney, A.B.; Waters, D.L.; Sinacore, D.R.; Colombo, E.; Armamento-Villareal, R.; Qualls, C. Aerobic or Resistance Exercise, or Both, in Dieting Obese Older Adults. *N. Engl. J. Med.* **2017**, *376*, 1943–1955. [CrossRef] [PubMed]
53. Alcazar, J.; Kamper, R.S.; Aagaard, P.; Haddock, B.; Prescott, E.; Ara, I.; Suetta, C. Relation between leg extension power and 30-s sit-to-stand muscle power in older adults: Validation and translation to functional performance. *Sci. Rep.* **2020**, *10*, 16337. [CrossRef] [PubMed]
54. Pulignano, G.; Del Sindaco, D.; Di Lenarda, A.; Alunni, G.; Senni, M.; Tarantini, L.; Cioffi, G.; Tinti, M.D.; Barbati, G.; Minardi, G.; et al. Incremental Value of Gait Speed in Predicting Prognosis of Older Adults With Heart Failure. *JACC Heart Fail.* **2016**, *4*, 289–298. [CrossRef]
55. Mercieca-Bebber, R.; King, M.T.; Calvert, M.J.; Stockler, M.R.; Friedlander, M. The importance of patient-reported outcomes in clinical trials and strategies for future optimization. *Patient Relat. Outcome Meas.* **2018**, *9*, 353–367. [CrossRef]

healthcare

MDPI

Review

Mechanical Efficiency and Injury Risk in Leg Kicks Across Combat Sports: A Narrative Review of Stance, Hip Rotation, and Striking Surface Effects

Soheil Sabri Razm [1], Kalenia Márquez-Flórez [2], Lucio Caprioli [3,*], Cristian Romagnoli [4,*], Saeid Edriss [3], Ida Cariati [5], Roberto Bonanni [4], Francesca Campoli [4], Virginia Tancredi [5], Elvira Padua [4] and Giuseppe Annino [1]

1 Human Performance Laboratory, Centre of Space Bio-Medicine, Department of Medicine Systems, University of Rome Tor Vergata, I-00133 Rome, Italy; soheil.sabrirazm@students.uniroma2.eu (S.S.R.); giuseppe.annino@uniroma2.it (G.A.)

2 Arts et Métiers Institute of Technology, EPF Engineering School, Université Sorbonne Paris Nord, IBHGC–Institut de Biomécanique HumaineGeorges Charpak, F-75013 Paris, France

3 Sports Engineering Laboratory, Department of Industrial Engineering, University of Rome Tor Vergata, I-00133 Rome, Italy; saeid.edriss@alumni.uniroma2.eu

4 Department of Human Science and Promotion of Quality of Life, San Raffaele Rome University, I-00166 Rome, Italy; roberto.bonanni@uniroma5.it (R.B.); francesca.campoli@uniroma5.it (F.C.); elvira.padua@uniroma5.it (E.P.)

5 Department of Systems Medicine, "Tor Vergata" University of Rome, Via Montpellier 1, I-00133 Rome, Italy; ida.cariati@uniroma2.it (I.C.); tancredi@uniroma2.it (V.T.)

* Correspondence: lucio.caprioli@uniroma2.it (L.C.); cristian.romagnoli@uniroma5.it (C.R.)

Highlights

What are the main findings?

- Pivot optimizes hip rotation and power but increases rotational stress on the knee and ankle of the supporting leg (risk of ACL and sprains).
- Contact with the tibia (shin) maximizes momentum but is associated with a high risk of tibial contusions and stress fractures (typical of Muay Thai/MMA).
- Contact with the instep promotes speed and scoring but exposes the foot and ankle to sprains and fractures.

What are the implications of the main findings?

- The same technical choices that maximize performance (impact force and speed) create specific vulnerabilities to injury.
- Results highlight a performance-safety continuum.

Abstract

Leg kicks are fundamental techniques in combat sports based on a proximal-distal sequence involving several factors that can affect mechanical efficiency and injury risk. However, there is a lack of comprehensive reviews that integrate biomechanical and epidemiological evidence on injuries in an interdisciplinary context. **Background/Objectives**: This narrative review synthesizes current evidence to explore the relationship between mechanical efficiency and injury risk in kick-based combat sports. **Methods**: The search was conducted across Web of Science and Scopus (January 2000–March 2025) or studies investigating the biomechanics and injury risk factors associated with leg kicks in Taekwondo, Karate, Muay Thai, Kickboxing, and MMA. **Results**: Analysis of 23 studies identified three primary technical determinants of efficiency: stance mechanics, hip rotation, and striking-surface selection. High-impact force is consistently associated with a pivoted support leg stance and proximal-to-distal coordination. However, these same mechanics create specific "load concentrations" that align with documented injury profiles: pivoted stances increase rotational stress on the support leg knee (ACL/meniscal strain), while striking-surface choice (shin vs. instep) dictates the trade-off between tibial stress and metatarsal/ankle trauma. **Conclusions**: This review proposes an Integrated mechanical efficiency–injury model that suggests that performance optimization and injury awareness are two sides of the same biomechanical process. Future research should fill the gaps relating to the subject's age and gender parity, as well as direct comparisons between different sports.

Keywords: kick biomechanics; taekwondo; stance stability; lower limb injuries; injury prevention; performance optimization

1. Introduction

Combat sports (CS) represent a variety of disciplines in which the human body is simultaneously an instrument of attack, a target, and a defense system, and in which there is often a subtle interaction between biomechanical principles and applied strategy [1,2]. In CS such as Muay Thai, Kickboxing, Mixed Martial Arts (MMA), Karate, and Taekwondo, leg kicks are fundamental techniques [3–5]. They serve key tactical functions, including disrupting opponents' balance, creating openings, and accumulating damage [6]. From a biomechanical perspective, effective leg kicking relies on proximal-to-distal sequencing, with stance, hip rotation, and striking surface selection being critical determinants for force transmission and postural stability [6–8]. These biomechanical characteristics influence both performance outcomes and injury mechanisms across CS.

Mechanical efficiency in martial arts kicking can be conceptualized as the ability to maximize mechanical output (e.g., foot velocity, joint angular velocity, impact force, or kinetic energy) relative to the neuromuscular and metabolic effort required, while minimizing energy losses due to unnecessary muscle co-contraction or inefficient movement coordination [9,10]. In general, high mechanical efficiency is achieved through the proximal-to-distal coordination of segmental motion, producing high distal segment velocities or impact energies without excessive muscle effort or compromising posture [11,12]. This concept is crucial as a biomechanical framework to compare kicking techniques across combat sports.

However, mechanical efficiency must be interpreted in light of the sport-specific constraints. What qualifies as an "effective" kick depends on the rules, tactical objectives, and scoring or impact criteria of each combat sport, which may prioritize speed, accuracy, contact force, or repeated execution [13,14]. Moreover, the biomechanical characteristics that might enhance performance may also increase musculoskeletal loading: pivoting may strain the support knee, shin contact may increase tibial stress, and instep striking may expose the foot to fractures [15–18]. Consequently, efficient kicking performance reflects a compromise between mechanical efficiency and injury risk, underscoring the need for integrative analyses that include both performance outcomes and injury mechanisms.

Existing literature on leg kicking remains largely fragmented and discipline-specific [19,20]. While such specialization is necessary given the specific characteristics of the different combat disciplines (technical, tactical, and constraining), it limits the comparison across CS and hinders the development of unified biomechanical principles of the efficacy and injury-free kicking. Hence, performance and injury outcomes are frequently examined in isolation or within a single sporting context.

This fragmentation is evident in the focus of performance-oriented studies; studies in Taekwondo emphasize speed and scoring-related variables [5,8], whereas research in Muay

 https://doi.org/10.3390/healthcare14040430

Thai or MMA prioritizes impact force and damage-related outcomes [4,18]. Injury surveillance studies show a similar sport-specific pattern, documenting foot and ankle injuries in instep-dominant sports [15,21] and shin or thigh trauma in shin-based styles [4,18]. The lack of a consistent methodological framework and common outcome measures complicates evidence synthesis, hides shared common performance and risk factors, and limits the translation of findings into cross-disciplinary training or injury-prevention strategies. Thus, studies integrating biomechanical and injury evidence to evaluate how stance, hip rotation, and strike-surface collectively influence both performance and injury risk across CS are lacking in the literature.

Previous reviews on kicking have been limited to specific disciplines, such as Taekwondo performance analyses or Karate injury epidemiology, without providing synthesis findings across different striking styles. To fill this gap, this review encompasses peer-reviewed studies published between January 2000 and March 2025, focusing on CS in which leg kicks are fundamental techniques. By combining evidence from biomechanics and sports medicine, the present study provides a cross-disciplinary synthesis aimed at advancing theoretical understanding, informing athlete preparation, and supporting injury prevention in combat sports. In line with the performance–injury framework outlined above, this review assumes that performance optimization and athlete safety should never be treated as separate goals but as interdependent aspects of high-level training and competition.

2. Materials and Methods

2.1. Eligibility

The inclusion criteria for this review were the following: (i) original articles published in English; (ii) studies published between January 2000 and March 2025; (iii) the population of the study was CS athletes, regardless of sex, age, or competitive level; (iv) athletes practicing CS in which leg kicks are fundamental (e.g., Muay Thai, Kickboxing, MMA, Karate, Taekwondo, Wushu); (v) studies reporting at least one biomechanical aspect (e.g., kinematic variables such as joint angles, angular velocities, and execution time; kinetic variables such as impact force, impulse, ground reaction forces, or joint moments; electromyographic activity or assessments of postural control and stability) or injury-related outcomes associated with leg kick execution; (vi) study designs including experimental, quasi-experimental, cross-sectional, prospective, or retrospective studies that reported primary data [22]. The exclusion criteria were as follows: (i) prospective studies or interventions not focused on CS, (ii) publications that did not correspond to original research (e.g., letters to the editor, translations, notes, and book reviews), (iii) case studies with one single athlete.

2.2. Information Sources and Search Strategy

A comprehensive literature search was conducted in the Web of Science Core Collection and Scopus databases, which are widely recognized as reliable sources for scientific publications [23,24].

The search strategy combined keywords related to leg kicks, biomechanics, injury, and combat sports, using Boolean operators to retrieve studies focused on kicking-related outcomes. It was performed within the Title, Abstract, and Keywords fields of the records. The search string was as follows: ("Mechanical efficiency" OR "Injury risk" OR "Leg kicks" OR "Hip rotation" OR "Stance" OR "Surface-strike") AND ("Combat Sport" OR "taekwondo" OR "martial arts" OR "karate" OR "MMA" OR "wushu" OR "muay Thai" OR "kickboxing").

 https://doi.org/10.3390/healthcare14040430

2.3. Study Selection and Data Extraction

All search results were exported fully recorded from Web of Science and Scopus datasets using Rayyan Software (Version 1.4.3). Duplicates across searches were systematically identified and removed using Digital Object Identifier (DOI) filtering. The remaining records were screened in three sequential stages.

(1) Title and Abstract Screening: Records clearly unrelated to combat sports, leg kicks, or biomechanics/injury outcomes (e.g., studies on Wrestling, Judo, or upper limb strikes) were excluded.
(2) Screening Groups: Each remaining record was categorized as "Included", "Excluded", or "Maybe". Studies in the "Maybe" category were not clearly irrelevant but required full-text review to determine eligibility.
(3) Full-Text Screening: Full texts were retrieved for all "Included" and "Maybe" articles. Studies that did not meet the eligibility criteria or were unavailable in full text were excluded.

2.4. Assessment of Methodological Quality

To evaluate the reliability of the findings from the included studies, the methodological quality of the included studies was assessed using a descriptive approach. However, given the narrative and integrative nature of this review and the significant heterogeneity in objectives, designs, and outcomes across studies, formal quantitative scoring and meta-analysis were not performed. Instead, this appraisal was used to contextualize the strength of the evidence, identify common methodological strengths and limitations across the literature, and inform the interpretation of the findings. The outcomes of this assessment are presented in Section 3.5.

2.5. Data Synthesis

For each included study, relevant data were extracted, analyzed, and registered into a standardized Excel spreadsheet, recording the following information: (i) author and year of publication; (ii) country of origin; (iii) combat sport; (iv) study design (experimental, cross-sectional, prospective, or retrospective); (v) sample: total number of participants, mean age, competitive level, and sex; (vi) biomechanical focus: stance mechanics, hip rotation, kinematic and kinetic variable; (vii) injury outcomes: injury type, prevalence, and mechanism; (viii) measurement tools; (ix) key findings.

3. Results

The initial search of the Web of Science and Scopus databases identified 282 records. After removing 61 duplicates, 40 non-English articles, and 24 records unrelated to CS or biomechanics, 154 records were retained for screening. Following title and abstract screening, 108 records were excluded for not meeting the inclusion criteria, leaving 46 reports sought for full-text retrieval. Of these, 24 reports were successfully retrieved, and 3 were excluded after full-text review (2 due to study design/comparator, 1 due to population not relevant). In addition to the database search, two relevant studies were identified through a forward manual searching of reference lists and included, as they matched the eligibility criteria previously described in Section 2.1. This resulted in a total of 23 studies included in the review. The study selection process is illustrated in the flowchart (Figure 1).

https://doi.org/10.3390/healthcare14040430

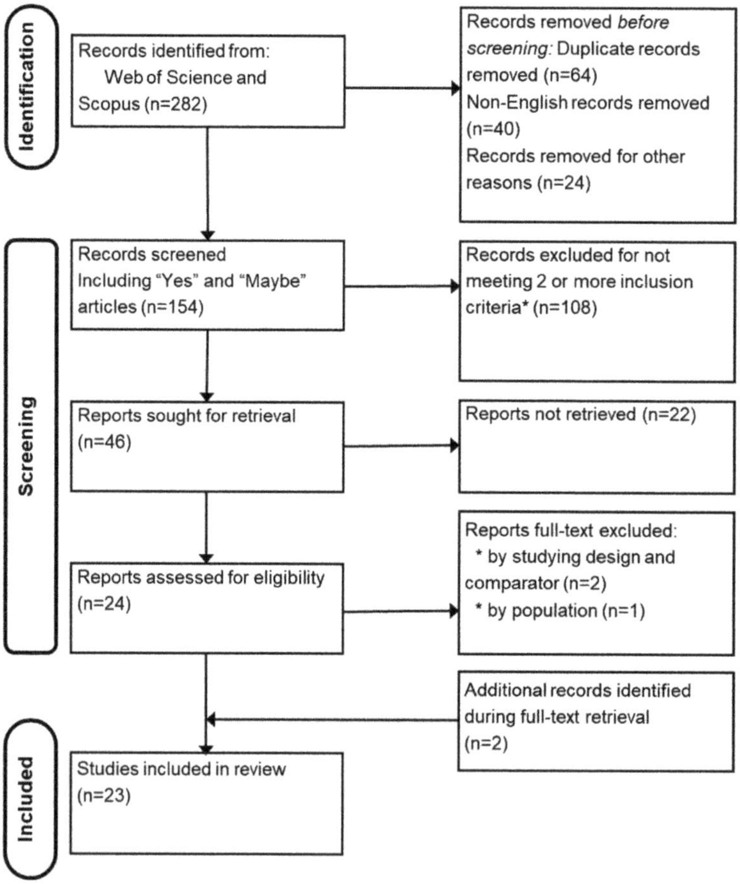

Figure 1. Flowchart of the review process. * Inclusion/Exclusion criteria described in the Materials and Methods section.

3.1. Characteristics of the Studies

The 23 included studies span Asia, Europe, North America, South America, and Oceania. Countries represented include Korea [7,17,19,25], Spain [8], the USA [4,15,26], Poland [27], Taiwan [7], Iran [28], Italy [5], the Czech Republic [6], Switzerland [20], Canada [3], Brazil [29], Australia [18], Ukraine [30], Romania [31], United Kingdom [32], Turkey [33], Australia [34], and multinational/international championship contexts [21]. Table 1 shows the summary of characteristics, effects, and variables analyzed in each selected study.

 https://doi.org/10.3390/healthcare14040430

Table 1. Characteristics and effects of studies about mechanical efficiency and injury risk in leg kicks across combat sports.

Study	Country	Combat Sport	Study Design	Sample	Biomechanical Focus	Injury Outcomes	Tools Used	Key Findings
Ramakrishnan et al., 2018 [26]	USA	Taekwondo	Experimental	n = 10 not specified	Kinetic variable: Energy transfer measurement	None	Force sensors	New method based on the force–time relation to quantify kick energy.
Park et al., 2021 [19]	Korea	Mixed Combat sports	Cross-sectional	n = 160 (m)	None	Injury prevalence (age)	Questionnaire	Injury risk increased with age, especially for lower limb injuries.
Zhao et al., 2022 [15]	USA	Taekwondo	Prospective	n = 183 m: 132 f: 41	None	Injury prevalence	Injury forms	In taekwondo, the lower limb is the most affected with high rates of ankle sprains and foot fractures.
Podrigalo et al., 2017 [30]	Ukraine	Martial Arts	Cross-sectional	n = 28 m: 20 f: 8	Hip rotation: Joint goniometry	None	Goniometer	Hip flexibility asymmetries are linked to kick efficiency.
Hsieh et al., 2012 [7]	Taiwan	Taekwondo	Experimental	n = 10 not specified	Hip rotation in a roundhouse kick	None	Motion capture	High hip rotation increases impact force and speed.
Kim et al., 2022 [16]	Korea	Taekwondo	Experimental	n = 20 m: 10 f: 10	Stance mechanics: ACL risk during pivot	Injury mechanism: risk modeling	Motion analysis	The pivoting leg shows high ACL stress in the supporting leg.
Daniel & Razvan, 2014 [31]	Romania	Karate	Experimental	n = 12 m: 10 f: 2	Stance mechanics: Plantar pressure vs. striking	None	Pressure plates	Higher plantar pressure correlated with stronger strikes.
Gorski & Orysiak, 2019 [27]	Poland	Taekwondo	Experimental	n = 16 (m)	Stance mechanics: Limb dominance in kicks	None	Force plates	Dominant leg kicking produced greater impact force.
Negahban et al., 2013 [28]	Iran	Taekwondo	Cross-sectional	n = 28 (m)	Stance mechanics: Postural control	None	Force plate	Taekwondo experts had better balance compared to shooting.
Everard et al., 2025 [32]	UK	Taekwondo	Prospective	n = 20 not specified	Stance mechanics	None	Motion capture	Stimulus cues improved performance, increasing speed and accuracy.

https://doi.org/10.3390/healthcare14040430

Table 1. *Cont.*

Study	Country	Combat Sport	Study Design	Sample	Biomechanical Focus	Injury Outcomes	Tools Used	Key Findings
Robbiani & Filippi, 2025 [20]	Switzerland	Muay Thai, K-1, Kickboxing	Cross-sectional	n = 325 m: 244 f: 81	None	Injury prevalence	Surveys	High motivation is linked with a higher injury rate.
Falco et al., 2009 [8]	Spain	Taekwondo	Experimental	n = 16 m: 12 f: 4	Kinetic: Kick distance	None	Force plates	A longer distance increased the force but slowed execution.
Lee et al., 2025 [17]	Korea	Taekwondo	Prospective	n = 98 m: 72 f: 26	None	Injury type	Monitoring logs	A high workload ratio increases injury incidence
Dong et al., 2025 [25]	Korea	Taekwondo	Cross-sectional	n = 40 m: 25 f: 15	kinetic	Injury prevalence	Isokinetic dynamometer and surveys	Muscle imbalance is linked to higher injury risk.
Zetaruk et al., 2000 [3]	USA	Karate	Retrospective	n = 263 m: 169 f: 94	None	Injury prevalence	Surveys	Most injuries were located in the lower limb, sprains being the most common.
Fares et al., 2019 [4]	USA	UFC (MMA)	Retrospective	n = 285 m: 249 f: 36	None	Injury prevalence and mechanisms	Medical records	Head injuries are the most common type of injury, followed by upper limb and lower limb injuries.
Strotmeyer & Lystad, 2017 [18]	Australia	Muay Thai	Cross-sectional	n = 136 m: 96 f: 40	None	Perceived risk	Surveys	Muay Thai fighters underestimate the risk of injury relative to other contact sports based on their own ability to negotiate risk.
Junior et al., 2025 [29]	Brazil	Muay Thai	Cross-sectional	n = 21 (m)	Kinetic	None	Heart rate variability monitor, Frequency speed of kick test	Heart rate variability, as an injury risk indicator, can be used by coaches to prevent injuries.

https://doi.org/10.3390/healthcare14040430

Table 1. *Cont.*

Study	Country	Combat Sport	Study Design	Sample	Biomechanical Focus	Injury Outcomes	Tools Used	Key Findings
Casolino et al., 2012 [5]	Italy	Taekwondo (Youth)	Cross-sectional	n = 24 not specified	Kinematic	None	Video analysis	Young athletes tend to use simpler techniques in competition, suggesting that coaches should emphasize coordination exercises to enhance performance.
Jandačka et al., 2013 [6]	Czechia	Taekwondo	Cross-sectional	n = 12 m: 6 f: 6	Stance mechanics	None	Force plates, movement capture analysis	The stance has little effect on kicking speed but a strong effect on hip power, which should be taken into account during training.
Augustovicova et al., 2019 [21]	International	Karate	Prospective	n = 778 m: 558 f: 220	None	Injury prevalence	*World Karate Federation* surveillance system	Only 10% injuries caused time loss, mainly due to upper-extremity fractures.
Doherty et al., 2025 [34]	Australia	MMA/Muay Thai	Prospective	n = 238 m: 180 f: 58	None	Injury prevalence	Questionnaire	High incidence of illness and injury during and after competition, with effects mainly limited to the 17 days post-competition.
Hallaçeli et al., 2025 [33]	Turkey	Muay Thai	Prospective	n = 663 m: 445 f: 218	None	Injury prevalence: Epidemiological analysis of athlete injuries	Direct Clinical Observation	Injury rates in official Muay Thai competition were low, likely due to medical supervision, protective equipment, and timely Referee Stop Contest (RSC) decisions, which help limit injury severity.

n: number of participants. m: number of male participants. f: number of female participants. TKD: taekwondo. ACL: anterior cruciate ligament. MMA: mixed martial arts. UFC: Ultimate Fighting Championship. Regarding combat sports, the majority of studies focused on Taekwondo (n = 12) [5–8,15–17,25–28,32], followed by Karate (n = 3) [3,21,31], Muay Thai/Kickboxing/K-1 (n = 5) [18,20,29,33,34], and Mixed Martial Arts/UFC (n = 4) [4,19,30,34].

https://doi.org/10.3390/healthcare14040430

In terms of study design, experimental biomechanical studies were the most frequent (n = 12) [5–8,16,25–29,31,32], while prospective or retrospective cohort designs were reported in five studies [3,4,15,17,21]. The remaining four employed cross-sectional or survey-based designs [18–20,30].

The vast majority of the 23 included studies fall into one of two distinct categories: controlled laboratory investigations of biomechanical efficiency (n = 13 experimental studies) or field-based observational reports of injury epidemiology (n = 12 prospective, retrospective, or cross-sectional studies). Notably, there are missing studies concurrently and prospectively measuring high-fidelity biomechanical variables (e.g., joint kinetics during a kick) and directly observing resultant injuries within the same cohort.

3.2. Sample Characteristics

Sample sizes ranged from laboratory-based cohorts (≈8–31 athletes) in biomechanics experiments [5–8,16,25,27–29,31,32] to large epidemiological surveillance datasets (hundreds of athlete exposures) [3,4,15,21]. Most biomechanical studies recruited competitive or elite athletes, particularly in Taekwondo [5–8,16,25,27,32], whereas epidemiological cohorts covered collegiate, national, and world-level competitions [15,17,21] as well as professional MMA/UFC events [4,34] and amateur Muay Thai/K-1/Kickboxing populations [18,20,29].

Sex distribution was male-dominant, though several studies included mixed-sex samples [3,5,15,20]. Age ranged from children/adolescents (e.g., Karate youth cohorts) [3,5] to adult amateurs and professionals in Muay Thai/K-1 [18,20,29,33,34] and collegiate/elite Taekwondo [6,8,15–17,25,32]. Across studies, common measurement approaches included 3D motion capture and force plates for mechanics [6–8,16,32], pressure platforms [31], impact sensors/dynamometry [8,26,27,29], isokinetic/balance testing [25], and medical/surveillance records or questionnaires for injury outcomes [3,4,15,17–19,21].

3.3. Mechanical Efficiency

Biomechanical studies consistently highlight the role of stance, hip rotation, and striking surface as the principal determinants of the mechanical efficiency of leg kicks across combat sports [7,8,29,31]. Objective measures, such as joint torques, ground-reaction forces, and postural control, suggest that efficient kicks require precise integration of balance and timing [28]. Athletes with superior postural control demonstrated greater accuracy and stability during unipedal stance [28].

Anthropometric characteristics also influenced performance outcomes, with longer limb segments and greater muscle mass generally associated with higher impact forces; however, intersegmental coordination remained the primary determinant of mechanical efficiency [27].

Overall, mechanical efficiency results from the coordination of stance mechanics, hip rotation, and striking surface choice. Stance sets the base for force transfer, hip rotation provides the primary engine of acceleration, and striking surface selection modulates the balance between power and speed [5–8,16,27,28,31].

3.4. Injury Outcomes

3.4.1. Anatomical Distribution

Injury data suggest that the lower extremities are the most commonly affected zones in combat sports [34]. The knee, ankle, shin, and foot are primary locations of injury, with the patterns influenced by the striking surface, stance mechanics, competitive context, and discipline. In Taekwondo, ankle sprains and foot fractures were frequently linked to instep kicking [8,15]. In shin-dominant striking disciplines, such as Muay Thai and kickboxing, tibial stress injuries were more common [18,20,33]. Additional injuries reported in Muay Thai included epistaxis, concussion, rib trauma, and extremity soft tissue strain.

 https://doi.org/10.3390/healthcare14040430

3.4.2. Incidence and Time-Loss Injuries

Prospective cohort studies in Taekwondo and Karate reported injury incidences ranging from 6–12 injuries per 1000 athlete exposures [15,21]. Surveys of MMA and Muay Thai competitors indicate that 39% of athletes reported at least one health problem, mostly superficial injuries (42.2%) and pain without specific tissue damage [34]. Observational studies during competition found that 91.4% of athletes experienced no health issues [33]. Time-loss injuries, defined as those preventing participation for one or more days, accounted for a substantial proportion of recorded cases, particularly at elite-level tournaments. In the World Karate Championships, approximately 10% of all reported injuries were classified as time loss, with fractures and joint sprains being the most disabling [21].

3.4.3. Mechanisms of Injury

Mechanistically, injuries arose both from attacking actions (e.g., excessive torsional stress on the support leg during pivoting) and receiving actions (e.g., blocked low kicks causing tibial or metatarsal trauma). Overuse injuries were reported less frequently and associated with high training loads, whereas acute traumatic injuries predominated during competition [3,15,21]. Training-related injuries were more often linked to cumulative workload and fatigue [17,29].

3.4.4. Risk Factors

Several studies identified risk modifiers that influenced injury occurrence. Higher acute-to-chronic workload ratios predicted lower-limb injury risk in Taekwondo [17]. Fatigue and autonomic imbalance, measured via heart rate variability in Muay Thai, were associated with greater susceptibility to injury [29]. Psychological and motivational factors also appeared relevant; athletes with higher competitive drive reported greater injury prevalence in Muay Thai, K-1, and Kickboxing [20].

3.5. Methodological Quality of Included Studies

The descriptive quality assessment revealed a pattern of methodological characteristics aligned with the two main research streams: controlled laboratory experiments and observational/epidemiological studies.

Laboratory-based biomechanical studies (n = 12) consistently demonstrated high internal validity for measuring discrete kinematic and kinetic parameters. The principal strengths were the use of objective and high-precision instrumentation (e.g., 3D motion capture, force plates) and standardized protocols. In this fragment, the main common limitations were small sample sizes (n < 30, often homogeneous in skill level), which reduced statistical power and generalizability; a focus on single-sport cohorts (predominantly Taekwondo); and the ecological validity of tasks, which may not fully replicate the cognitive and tactical demands of competition.

Observational injury studies (n = 11) provided valuable data on incidence and mechanisms in real-world settings. Prospective designs with active surveillance at competitions offered the most reliable injury data. Common limitations included: variability in injury definitions and reporting methods across studies, which complicates comparison; potential for recall and selection bias in survey-based and retrospective designs; and, in many cases, a lack of adjustment for key confounders such as training load, prior injury history, or protective equipment use.

Notably, only a minority of studies integrated biomechanical and injury outcomes within the same research framework. This methodological divide underscores the core challenge addressed by this review: synthesizing evidence from high-control/low-ecology

https://doi.org/10.3390/healthcare14040430

experiments with low-control/high-ecology observational data to form a coherent understanding of the performance–injury relationship.

The substantial heterogeneity in outcome measures and data collection methodologies across studies is a notable challenge in synthesizing the evidence, limiting direct comparability. To clarify this heterogeneity, the biomechanical and clinical measures employed in the included literature are categorized and presented, along with their primary limitations, in Supplementary Table S1.

4. Discussion

This review included 23 studies spanning Taekwondo, Karate, Muay Thai/K-1/Kickboxing, and MMA, integrating biomechanical and injury-related evidence on leg kicks. Across the studies, three technical determinants consistently emerged as primary drivers of mechanical efficiency: stance/support leg mechanics, hip rotation/sequencing, and striking surface selection [5–8,16,27,28,31]. Injury surveillance consistently identified the lower extremity—particularly the ankle, knee, shin, and foot—as the most frequent and consequential sites of injury in striking contexts [3,4,8,15,17,18,20,21,29]. When these streams are combined, a pattern emerges: the same technical features that enhance efficiency also create load concentrations and tissue-specific injury risk.

4.1. Biomechanical Paradox

The core finding of this review is that mechanical efficiency and injury risk are not independent variables; rather, the technical features that optimize impact force are the same features that lead to important loads on musculoskeletal tissues.

4.1.1. Stance Mechanics and the Pivot "Penalty"

Stance emerged as a key determinant of force generation, transfer, and stability. Orthogonal or pivoted support leg position, like in Taekwondo, facilitated greater hip rotation and joint power, improving impact potential, whereas non-pivoted or narrower stances limited force transfer and balance [6,8,16]. However, this mechanical advantage comes with a "penalty." Pivoted stances increase rotational stress on the knee and tibia of the supporting leg, aligning with ACL-relevant loading. This explains the high incidence of ACL and meniscal injuries found in surveillance data [13,15,19]. Mechanical efficiency in this context is a trade-off between force transfer and joint preservation.

4.1.2. Hip Rotation and Force–Risk Trade-Offs

In general, the hip acts as the biomechanical "engine" of leg kicks. Higher pelvic/hip angular velocity improved to peak impact force and execution speed when the timing along the thigh–shank–foot chain was maintained [7,8]. In fact, proximal-to-distal sequencing—i.e., rotational momentum generated proximally and released distally—was confirmed as critical for efficient impulse transfer, with longer approach distances allowing greater hip acceleration but slower time to contact [7,8,16,32]. However, rapid pelvic acceleration propagated higher rotational and shear loads through the kinetic chain, increasing stress concentrations at the support knee and distal striking surface [8,16]. This suggests that athletes who maximize hip torque for performance may be placing their joints under repetitive high-strain cycles that lead to chronic stress and fatigue-related injuries noted in elite cohorts.

4.2. Contact Mechanics and Striking Surface

The choice of striking surface represents the most direct performance–risk compromise identified in the literature. Each strike-surface choice, therefore, reflects a biomechanical compromise between efficiency and injury exposure.

 https://doi.org/10.3390/healthcare14040430

Force-Speed Trade-Off

Force-oriented disciplines, such as Muay Thai, prefer the shin as a striking surface [5,8,27,32] because it provides higher impulse transfer and stiffer contact mechanics, maximizing impact force [5,27]. Nevertheless, shin contact enhances the onset of tibial contusions/stress injuries [18,20], periosteal stress, and quadriceps bruising [4,18,20]. Conversely, speed-oriented disciplines (e.g., Taekwondo) favorize instep strikes as they allow for increased strike velocity and scoring speed at the cost of lower force [8,32]. While this improves scoring potential, the smaller bone structures and higher distal velocities lead to the high risk of fractures and sprains documented in these populations [3,5,8,15,18,20,27].

4.3. *Modifiers: Anthropometry, Fatigue, and Psychology*

These trade-offs can be modulated by the individual characteristics of the athlete. Indeed, in the actualization of this potential, individual and psychosocial factors play their decisive role [35]. An athlete's motivational drive and cultural framing act as a gain control, amplifying or attenuating the consistent application of high-risk, high-efficiency techniques in training and competition, thereby directly influencing injury epidemiology [36].

4.3.1. Anthropometry

While longer limbs or greater lean mass can result in a larger moment arm for higher impact forces [25], this can also mean a greater moment force is applied to the joints at a given instant, as when the kick is blocked. Additionally, coordination/timing performance relies deeply on the morphology of the individual [27]. This could suggest that the overall anthropometry of the athlete determines the speed and force produced by the subject.

4.3.2. Fatigue

Fatigue can influence the transition from an efficient strike to an injurious one. With the alteration of the balance between agonist and antagonist muscles and the consequent decline in neuromuscular control [28] due to fatigue, kicking efficiency is reduced, and thus even a technically correct kick could become a high-risk event [17,29]. In other words, the neuromuscular system's ability to reduce the stress on the joints through proper muscle coactivation is compromised. This is more risky in young cohorts, as less mature neuromuscular control is particularly vulnerable to imbalance between performance goals and tissue tolerance [3,25].

4.3.3. Perceived Versus Actual Risk

As studies have shown [18], injury is often viewed as an inherent component of combat sports. This makes the athletes prioritize performance (e.g., impact force or speed) over joint preservation. While athletes might perceive the injuries of the striking surface as the primary threat—leading to a psychological focus on shin conditioning—they often lack a corresponding concern for the support leg's ligamentous safety [18]. This creates a false perception of the athlete where the most dangerous mechanics are the least feared.

Moreover, evidence from Muay Thai and Kickboxing [20] indicates that high competitive drive and motivational orientation are significant predictors of injury prevalence. Athletes with higher drive tend to misinterpret or ignore physiological signals of fatigue and autonomic imbalance [20]. This drive–risk relationship might suggest that the psychological commitment to efficiency often overrides the biological warning systems intended to prevent tissue failure.

4.3.4. Gender Dimorphism

Anatomical, hormonal, and neuromuscular dimorphisms suggest plausible ways in which the proposed efficiency–injury model components might be differentially expressed

https://doi.org/10.3390/healthcare14040430

or modulated in female athletes. The typically wider quadriceps angle (Q-angle) in females alters the alignment of the patellofemoral joint and the force vector of the quadriceps on the tibia [37]. During a pivoted kick, this could theoretically increase lateral patellar shear and exacerbate the rotational stress on the supporting ACL [38,39]. Also, fluctuations in estrogen across the menstrual cycle may change ligament laxity and collagen synthesis [40,41], lowering the load threshold at which ligaments succumb to the torsional and shear forces generated during the kicks.

4.4. Practical Implications

The synthesis of biomechanical efficiency, injury epidemiology, and psychological risk factors suggests that performance and injury prevention in combat sports are linked. Hence, the following targeted interventions are proposed.

4.4.1. For Coaches and Technical Staff

Coaches should recognize the stance/pivot high-performance/risk mechanics [6,8,16,17]. Hence, coaches should treat it as a specialized skill. Technical practice should therefore emphasize controlled pivot execution and progressive loading of support leg stability to minimize torsional knee stress, for example, practice kicks starting with a minimal pivot (e.g., 30°), focusing on stability, then gradually increasing the rotation angle as control improves.

Moreover, coaches should train athletes to match their striking surface to the discipline context. For instance, using the shin for high-power, low-speed delivery (Muay Thai/MMA) requires specific bone-loading conditioning, whereas instep strikes in scoring-based sports (Taekwondo/Karate) require specific ankle stabilization exercises to prevent fractures [3,15,18,20,21]. Coaches should actively target supplemental training based on the discipline's dominant risks. If relying on pivoted kicks, prioritizing single-leg stability, Bulgarian split squat [42], eccentric hamstring strength (e.g., Nordic curls), and Romanian deadlift [43] in gym work can protect the support knee [44]. Focusing on ankle strengthening (e.g., banded eversions) and foot arch exercises (short-foot drills, marble pickups) for strikes with the instep is also beneficial.

Technical staff should work to decouple the normalization of risk from high performance by recognizing that a very motivated athlete [20] is likely to hide fatigue and pain. Hence, coaches should use objective measures (e.g., kick speed drop-off or heart rate variability) rather than athlete self-reporting to determine the training volume.

4.4.2. For Athletes

Athletes should be educated on the performance–risk trade-offs of technical choices. Developing bilateral proficiency in stance and striking surface may diversify tactical options and distribute loading more evenly across limbs. They should actively engage in targeted supplemental training based on their discipline's dominant risks. Workload monitoring, including acute-to-chronic training ratios, should be adopted to reduce overuse and fatigue-related injuries [17,29]. Regular balance and proprioceptive training may mitigate the instability that predisposes athletes to support leg injuries [25,28].

4.4.3. For Clinicians and Sports Medicine Practitioners

Clinical screening for strength and balance asymmetries (e.g., between dominant and non-dominant legs) can identify athletes at elevated risk [25]. Rehabilitation should address both the injured tissue and the mechanical chain (e.g., retraining hip control after ankle injury, or support leg stability after knee injury). Injury surveillance systems in competition and training should distinguish between instep, shin, and knee-related injuries, enabling more precise risk monitoring [3,4,15,18,20,21].

https://doi.org/10.3390/healthcare14040430

When treating an injured combat athlete, clinicians should assess their "Competitive Drive" [20]. High-drive athletes may require more rigid return-to-play protocols to prevent them from returning too early due to an underestimated perception of risk.

4.5. Future Directions

While the current literature mentions the basic knowledge of leg kicks, several critical gaps remain. Future research should prioritize the following four areas to move the field toward a more predictive and preventive science.

The majority of studies recruited predominantly male participants, with limited attention to female athletes or youth cohorts. Future work should conduct sex-disaggregated analyses of biomechanical efficiency and injury risk, as sex-related differences in joint laxity, neuromuscular control, and injury profiles are well documented in other sports [38]. Similarly, research should focus on adolescent development phases, where imbalances in growth, coordination, and strength may exacerbate injury vulnerability [3,25].

Training load ratios are linked to injury outcomes [17,29], yet most studies were short-term or cross-sectional. Future research should employ longitudinal cohort designs that track athletes across training cycles and competitive seasons, enabling clearer identification of workload thresholds associated with injury onset. Integration of injury surveillance with biomechanical testing would allow direct mapping of mechanical efficiency metrics onto long-term health outcomes.

Research is needed to evaluate the effectiveness of prevention strategies—for example, proprioceptive training, stance-modification drills, and tibial/ankle conditioning—on both reducing injury incidence and maintaining performance outcomes. Such interventions should be tested in collaboration with coaches, clinicians, and athletes, ensuring feasibility in real-world training contexts.

Although this review included Taekwondo, Karate, Muay Thai, Kickboxing, and MMA, the evidence base remains skewed toward Taekwondo. Future studies should expand direct biomechanical comparisons across sports. Such cross-sport analyses could clarify how rule sets and coaching traditions shape the efficiency–injury continuum.

Advances in wearable sensors, inertial measurement units (IMUs) [45], and machine learning analytics [46,47] provide opportunities for more ecological measurements [48–50]. Future studies should leverage these technologies to validate laboratory findings in ecological, training, and competitive environments. This would support data-driven feedback systems for both performance enhancement and injury prevention.

A link between competitive drive, fatigue, and injury was found [18,20]. Future research should adopt a multivariate approach. Integrating biomechanical metrics (e.g., peak hip velocity) with psychological assessments (e.g., risk perception scales) and physiological data (e.g., Heart Rate Variability) would allow researchers to create a "Risk Profile" for individual athletes. This could lead to machine learning models [46,47] capable of predicting injury windows based on the interaction of technical output and psychological state.

Ultimately, the goal should be to develop predictive, quantitative models that can estimate injury probability for a given athlete based on the weighted inputs of their biomechanical technique, physiological readiness, and psychosocial profile (e.g., score on risk-taking propensity scales) [51]. This would move the field from descriptive frameworks to actionable, personalized risk assessment.

Few controlled experiments directly compared shin vs. instep striking, or pivot vs. non-pivot stances, under standardized conditions. Randomized, lab-based trials examining these variations could establish causal links between technique, mechanical efficiency, and injury mechanisms, strengthening the biomechanical–epidemiological synthesis.

 https://doi.org/10.3390/healthcare14040430

Beyond combat sports, these findings contribute to broader sports biomechanics by illustrating how technique sequencing interacts with injury mechanisms in dynamic striking tasks. The efficiency–injury trade-off model may therefore inform not only martial arts training but also sports medicine approaches to activities with similar rotational loading, such as soccer kicking [52], tennis [53–55], or hockey shooting [56,57].

4.6. Strengths and Limitations

The principal strength of this review lies in its cross-disciplinary synthesis. By integrating biomechanical and injury evidence on leg kicks, this review provides a unified framework that moves beyond the typical "lab vs. clinic" divide. Hence, this review highlights the direct overlap between performance determinants and injury mechanisms, offering a unified framework relevant to athletes, coaches, and clinicians. Previous research streams have tended to isolate either mechanical efficiency (laboratory biomechanics) or injury incidence (epidemiology and surveillance).

The inclusion of diverse CS (Taekwondo, Karate, Muay Thai, Kickboxing, MMA) further strengthens the generalizability of the findings across striking-based disciplines. However, discipline distribution was uneven, with Taekwondo being disproportionately represented relative to other sports, such as Muay Thai and MMA, which are underrepresented. This gives more weight to instep-dominant sports, potentially biasing the synthesis toward rule sets emphasizing speed and scoring efficiency. This limitation may bias the outcomes; therefore, future studies should consider conducting larger, separate analyses by discipline.

Several other limitations should temper interpretation. First, sex representation was uneven, with the majority of included participants being male. Only a minority of studies provided sex-disaggregated analyses, limiting the applicability of findings to female athletes. Second, sample sizes in biomechanics experiments were generally small (often fewer than 20 participants), which constrains statistical power and the representativeness of mechanical efficiency findings. Third, heterogeneity in measurement approaches—including motion capture systems, force sensors, and injury surveillance protocols—limited direct comparability of outcomes across studies. The narrative and integrative nature of this review, necessitated by the heterogeneity in designs, populations, and measures described above, means that its findings should be interpreted as hypothesis-generating rather than as definitive conclusions. Furthermore, because current data are mostly based on tests performed in the laboratory, there is a need for future longitudinal studies that collect data in real-time sparring environments using wearable sensors (e.g., IMUs) and video systems. Taking care that the protocol of using wearable sensors must be followed in practical exercises on a single player, avoiding contact with another participant.

Finally, the main search relied solely on the Web of Science Core Collection and Scopus, excluding relevant literature indexed in other sources (e.g., PubMed, SPORTDiscus), which substantially increased the risk of publication bias and limited the comprehensiveness of the included evidence. In addition, no manual backward or forward reference searching was systematically performed beyond these sources, and it may have excluded relevant studies indexed elsewhere.

5. Conclusions

This review proposes and synthesizes evidence supporting the concept that mechanical efficiency and injury risk in leg kicks across combat sports are inseparable. The technical determinants of a powerful strike—specifically the pivoted stance and proximal-to-distal hip sequencing—appear to be closely associated with the same mechanisms that generate hazardous loads on the support leg knee and striking surface. Pivoted stances and rapid hip

 https://doi.org/10.3390/healthcare14040430

rotation enhance impact force and timing but elevate knee loading; shin strikes maximize impulse transfer but predispose athletes to tibial trauma; and instep strikes facilitate speed yet expose the foot and ankle to fractures and sprains.

By connecting laboratory biomechanics with epidemiological evidence, this review constructs a performance–safety continuum that offers a plausible explanatory framework for why efficiency gains frequently coincide with injury vulnerabilities. The framework suggests practical guidance for athletes, coaches, and clinicians: technical refinement, load monitoring, and targeted conditioning can balance the trade-offs between maximizing performance and minimizing risk. However, considering the connections between kinematic parameters, joint and tissue stress are drawn from a fragmented evidence base where biomechanical cause and injury effect are rarely measured in conjunction.

Supplementary Materials: The following supporting information can be downloaded at: https://www.mdpi.com/article/10.3390/healthcare14040430/s1, Table S1: Categorization of outcome measures and their methodological considerations in studies on leg kick biomechanics and injury.

Author Contributions: Conceptualization, S.S.R., L.C., C.R. and G.A.; methodology, S.S.R., L.C., K.M.-F., C.R. and G.A.; formal analysis, S.S.R.; investigation, S.S.R.; resources, S.S.R.; data curation, S.S.R.; writing—original draft preparation, S.S.R., L.C. and C.R.; writing—review and editing, L.C., K.M.-F., C.R., S.E., I.C., R.B. and F.C.; visualization, V.T. and E.P.; supervision, K.M.-F., V.T., E.P. and G.A. All authors have read and agreed to the published version of the manuscript.

Funding: This research received no external funding.

Institutional Review Board Statement: Not applicable.

Informed Consent Statement: Not applicable.

Data Availability Statement: No new data were created or analyzed in this study. Data sharing is not applicable to this article.

Conflicts of Interest: The authors declare no conflicts of interest.

Abbreviations

The following abbreviations are used in this manuscript:

CS	Combat Sports
ACL	Anterior Cruciate Ligament
MMA	Mixed Martial Arts
DOI	Digital Object Identifier
WKF	World Karate Federation
UFC	Ultimate Fighting Championship
TKD	Taekwondo

References

1. Miarka, B.; Brito, C.J.; Moreira, D.G.; Amtmann, J. Differences by Ending Rounds and Other Rounds in Time-Motion Analysis of Mixed Martial Arts: Implications for Assessment and Training. *J. Strength Cond. Res.* **2018**, *32*, 534–544. [CrossRef]
2. Górski, M.; Kubacki, R.; Buśko, K. Comparison of Muscle Strength Profiles in Taekwondo and Judo Elite Athletes. *Acta Bioeng. Biomech.* **2025**, *26*, 79–88. [CrossRef]
3. Zetaruk, M.N.; Violan, M.A.; Zurakowski, D.; Micheli, L.J. Karate Injuries in Children and Adolescents. *Accid. Anal. Prev.* **2000**, *32*, 421–425. [CrossRef]
4. Fares, M.Y.; Fares, J.; Fares, Y.; Abboud, J.A. Musculoskeletal and Head Injuries in the Ultimate Fighting Championship (UFC). *Physician Sportsmed.* **2019**, *47*, 205–211. [CrossRef]
5. Casolino, E.; Lupo, C.; Cortis, C.; Chiodo, S.; Minganti, C.; Capranica, L.; Tessitore, A. Technical and Tactical Analysis of Youth Taekwondo Performance. *J. Strength Cond. Res.* **2012**, *26*, 1489–1495. [CrossRef] [PubMed]

 https://doi.org/10.3390/healthcare14040430

6. Jandačka, D.; Estevan, I.; Janura, M.; Falco, C. The Impact of the Initial Stance Position on Lower Limb Joint Kinetics in the Taekwondo Roundhouse Kick. *Acta Gymnica* **2013**, *43*, 15–22. [CrossRef]
7. Hsieh, A.; Huang, C.-F.; Huang, C.C. The Biomechanical Analysis of Roundhouse Kick in Taekwondo. In *Proceedings of the ISBS-Conference Proceedings Archive*; International Society of Biomechanics in Sports (ISBS): Melbourne, Australia, 2012.
8. Falco, C.; Alvarez, O.; Castillo, I.; Estevan, I.; Martos, J.; Mugarra, F.; Iradi, A. Influence of the Distance in a Roundhouse Kick's Execution Time and Impact Force in Taekwondo. *J. Biomech.* **2009**, *42*, 242–248. [CrossRef]
9. Hagler, S. Patterns of Selection of Human Movements IV: Energy Efficiency, Mechanical Advantage, and Asynchronous Arm-Cranking. *arXiv* **2017**, arXiv:1702.03271.
10. Romagnoli, C.; Caprioli, L.; Cariati, I.; Campoli, F.; Edriss, S.; Frontuto, C.; Galvan, A.; Giugliano, M.; Martinez, E.R.; Padua, E.; et al. Use of an IMU Device to Assess the Performance in Swimming and Match Positions of Impaired Water Polo Athletes: A Pilot Study. *Appl. Sci.* **2025**, *15*, 8826. [CrossRef]
11. Vagner, M.; Cleather, D.J.; Olah, V.; Vacek, J.; Stastny, P. A Systematic Review of Dynamic Forces and Kinematic Indicators of Front and Roundhouse Kicks across Varied Conditions and Participant Experience. *Sports* **2023**, *11*, 141. [CrossRef]
12. Verrelli, C.M.; Caprioli, L.; Iosa, M. Hidden Time-Patterns in Cyclic Human Movements: A Matter of Temporal Fibonacci Sequence Generation and Harmonization. *Front. Hum. Neurosci.* **2025**, *19*, 1525403. [CrossRef] [PubMed]
13. Diniz, R.; Del Vecchio, F.B.; Schaun, G.Z.; Oliveira, H.B.; Portella, E.G.; Da Silva, E.S.; Formalioni, A.; Campelo, P.C.; Peyré-Tartaruga, L.A.; Pinto, S.S. Kinematic Comparison of the Roundhouse Kick between Taekwondo, Karate, and Muaythai. *J. Strength Cond. Res.* **2021**, *35*, 198–204. [CrossRef] [PubMed]
14. Gavagan, C.J.; Sayers, M.G. A Biomechanical Analysis of the Roundhouse Kicking Technique of Expert Practitioners: A Comparison between the Martial Arts Disciplines of Muay Thai, Karate, and Taekwondo. *PLoS ONE* **2017**, *12*, e0182645. [CrossRef]
15. Zhao, R.T.; Medina, G.; Chen, E.T.; Oh, L.S. Acute Injuries in American Collegiate Taekwondo Competitions: A Prospective Study Spanning Four Competitive Seasons. *J. Sports Med. Phys. Fit.* **2022**, *62*, 517–524. [CrossRef]
16. Kim, K.; Davaasambuu, B.; Wei, R.; Kim, Y.H. Biomechanical Investigation of Anterior Cruciate Ligament Injury Risk in Pivoting Leg during Taekwondo Kicks Using Motion Analysis System. *J. Mech. Sci. Technol.* **2022**, *36*, 1051–1056. [CrossRef]
17. Lee, J.; Lim, J.; Kim, S.; Song, I.; Lim, S.; Yoon, J.; Park, J. Injury Incidences Related to Acute-to-Chronic Workload Ratios in Taekwondo: A Prospective Study with a 3-Year Follow-Up. *J. Athl. Train.* **2025**, *60*, 569–576. [CrossRef]
18. Strotmeyer, S., Jr.; Lystad, R.P. Perception of Injury Risk among Amateur Muay Thai Fighters. *Inj. Epidemiol.* **2017**, *4*, 2. [CrossRef]
19. Park, S.; Kim, Y.; Woo, S.; Lee, O. A Survey Study on Sports Injury by Age for Male Athletes in Combat Sports. *J. Men's Health* **2021**, *17*, 120–126.
20. Robbiani, A.I.; Filippi, A. From Fitness to Fight: Associations between Training Motivation and Injury Prevalence in Muay Thai, K-1 and Kickboxing: Results of a Nationwide Swiss Survey. *SWISS Dent. J. SSO–Sci. Clin. Top.* **2025**, *135*, 62–71. [CrossRef]
21. Augustovičová, D.; Lystad, R.P.; Arriaza, R. Time-Loss Injuries in Karate: A Prospective Cohort Study of 4 Consecutive World Karate Championships. *Orthop. J. Sports Med.* **2019**, *7*, 2325967119865866. [CrossRef] [PubMed]
22. Lefebvre, C.; Glanville, J.; Briscoe, S.; Littlewood, A.; Marshall, C.; Metzendorf, M.-I.; Noel-Storr, A.; Rader, T.; Shokraneh, F.; Thomas, J.; et al. Searching for and Selecting Studies. In *Cochrane Handbook for Systematic Reviews of Interventions*; John Wiley & Sons: Hoboken, NJ, USA, 2019; pp. 67–107.
23. Falagas, M.E.; Pitsouni, E.I.; Malietzis, G.A.; Pappas, G. Comparison of PubMed, Scopus, Web of Science, and Google Scholar: Strengths and Weaknesses. *FASEB J.* **2008**, *22*, 338–342. [CrossRef]
24. Chadegani, A.A.; Salehi, H.; Yunus, M.M.; Farhadi, H.; Fooladi, M.; Farhadi, M.; Ebrahim, N.A. A Comparison between Two Main Academic Literature Collections: Web of Science and Scopus Databases. *arXiv* **2013**, arXiv:1305.0377. [CrossRef]
25. Dong, M.; Kim, B.; Lee, J.; Choi, Y.; Shi, P.; Zhang, G. Isokinetic Muscle Function, Dynamic Balance, and Injury Risk in Dominant and Non-Dominant Lower Extremities of Adolescent Taekwondo Athletes. *Front. Sports Act. Living* **2025**, *7*, 1599516. [CrossRef] [PubMed]
26. Ramakrishnan, K.R.; Wang, H.; Shankar, K.; Fien, A. A New Method for the Measurement and Analysis of Biomechanical Energy Delivered by Kicking. *Sports Eng.* **2018**, *21*, 53–62. [CrossRef]
27. Górski, M.; Orysiak, J. Differences between Anthropometric Indicators and the Impact Force of Taekwondo Kicks Performed with the Dominant and Non-Dominant Limb. *Biomed. Hum. Kinet.* **2019**, *11*, 193–197. [CrossRef]
28. Negahban, H.; Aryan, N.; Mazaheri, M.; Norasteh, A.A.; Sanjari, M.A. Effect of Expertise in Shooting and Taekwondo on Bipedal and Unipedal Postural Control Isolated or Concurrent with a Reaction-Time Task. *Gait Posture* **2013**, *38*, 226–230. [CrossRef]
29. Junior, A.B.D.A.; De Andrade, E.M.; Vigário, P.D.S.; Luchesa, C.A.; Vieira, J.E.D.A.; De Jesus, I.R.; Lopes, A.J. Relationships Between Performance in the Frequency Speed Kick Test, Heart Rate Variability, and Body Composition in Amateur Muay Thai Fighters. *Int. J. Exerc. Sci.* **2025**, *18*, 428. [CrossRef]
30. Podrigalo, L.; Volodchenko, A.; Rovnaya, O.; Stankiewicz, B. Analysis of Martial Arts Athletes' Goniometric Indicators. *Phys. Educ. Stud.* **2017**, *21*, 182–188. [CrossRef]

 https://doi.org/10.3390/healthcare14040430

31. Daniel, T.M.; Răzvan-Liviu, P. Correlation between Plantar Pressure and Striking Speed in Karate-Do. *Procedia-Soc. Behav. Sci.* **2014**, *117*, 357–360. [CrossRef]
32. Everard, S.; Chang, M.; Landeo, R. Enhancing Taekwondo Performance: The Role of Pre-Kicking Techniques and Stimulus Triggers in Elite Athletes. *J. Sports Sci.* **2025**, *43*, 1036–1043. [CrossRef] [PubMed]
33. Hallaçeli, H.; Davut, S.; Özbek, A.; Aydın, E. Epidemiological Analysis of Athlete Injuries in Muay Thai In-Ring Matches. *Inj. Epidemiol.* **2025**, *12*, 28. [CrossRef]
34. Doherty, C.S.; Barley, O.R.; Fortington, L.V. Incidence of Health Problems in Australian Mixed Martial Arts and Muay Thai Competitors: A 14-Month Study of 26 Combat Sports Events. *Sports Med.-Open* **2025**, *11*, 60. [CrossRef]
35. Bae, M. Biopsychosocial Approach to Sports Injury: A Systematic Review and Exploration of Knowledge Structure. *BMC Sports Sci. Med. Rehabil.* **2024**, *16*, 242. [CrossRef]
36. Ivarsson, A.; Johnson, U.; Andersen, M.B.; Tranaeus, U.; Stenling, A.; Lindwall, M. Psychosocial Factors and Sport Injuries: Meta-Analyses for Prediction and Prevention. *Sports Med.* **2017**, *47*, 353–365. [CrossRef]
37. Gant, H.; Ghimire, N.; Min, K.; Musa, I.; Ashraf, M.; Lawan, A. Impact of the Quadriceps Angle on Health and Injury Risk in Female Athletes. *Int. J. Environ. Res. Public Health* **2024**, *21*, 1547. [CrossRef] [PubMed]
38. Gianakos, A.L.; Hartman, H.; Kerkhoffs, G.M.; Calder, J.; Kennedy, J.G. Sex Differences in Biomechanical Properties of the Achilles Tendon May Predispose Men to Higher Risk of Injury: A Systematic Review. *J. ISAKOS* **2024**, *9*, 184–191. [CrossRef] [PubMed]
39. Hewett, T.E.; Myer, G.D.; Ford, K.R. Anterior Cruciate Ligament Injuries in Female Athletes: Part 1, Mechanisms and Risk Factors. *Am. J. Sports Med.* **2006**, *34*, 299–311. [CrossRef]
40. Shultz, S.J.; Fegley, J.A. The Effect of Sex Hormones on Ligament Structure, Joint Stability and ACL Injury Risk. In *Sex Hormones, Exercise and Women: Scientific and Clinical Aspects*; Springer: Berlin/Heidelberg, Germany, 2023; pp. 167–195.
41. Gilmer, G.; Crasta, N.; Tanaka, M.J. The Effect of Sex Hormones on Joint Ligament Properties: A Systematic Review and Meta-Analysis. *Am. J. Sports Med.* **2025**, *53*, 2738–2748. [CrossRef]
42. Mackey, E.R.; Riemann, B.L. Biomechanical Differences between the Bulgarian Split-Squat and Back Squat. *Int. J. Exerc. Sci.* **2021**, *14*, 533. [CrossRef] [PubMed]
43. McAllister, M.J.; Hammond, K.G.; Schilling, B.K.; Ferreria, L.C.; Reed, J.P.; Weiss, L.W. Muscle Activation during Various Hamstring Exercises. *J. Strength Cond. Res.* **2014**, *28*, 1573–1580. [CrossRef]
44. Van Dyk, N.; Pecci, J. May the (Horizontal) Force Be with You: The Role of Ankle Function and Horizontal Force Production on Hamstring Injury Risk and Rehabilitation. *Br. J. Sports Med.* **2025**, *59*, 1332–1334. [CrossRef]
45. Pezenka, L.; Wirth, K. Reliability of a Low-Cost Inertial Measurement Unit (IMU) to Measure Punch and Kick Velocity. *Sensors* **2025**, *25*, 307. [CrossRef]
46. Zanela, A.; Caprioli, L.; Frontuto, C.; Bonaiuto, V. Integrative Analysis of Movement: AI-Enhanced Video and Inertial Sensors in Athletic Contexts. In *Proceedings of the International Workshop on Engineering Methodologies for Medicine and Sport*; Springer: Berlin/Heidelberg, Germany, 2024; pp. 625–641.
47. Cizmic, D.; Hoelbling, D.; Baranyi, R.; Breiteneder, R.; Grechenig, T. Smart Boxing Glove "RD α": IMU Combined with Force Sensor for Highly Accurate Technique and Target Recognition Using Machine Learning. *Appl. Sci.* **2023**, *13*, 9073. [CrossRef]
48. Edriss, S.; Romagnoli, C.; Caprioli, L.; Zanela, A.; Panichi, E.; Campoli, F.; Padua, E.; Annino, G.; Bonaiuto, V. The Role of Emergent Technologies in the Dynamic and Kinematic Assessment of Human Movement in Sport and Clinical Applications. *Appl. Sci.* **2024**, *14*, 1012. [CrossRef]
49. Edriss, S.; Romagnoli, C.; Caprioli, L.; Bonaiuto, V.; Padua, E.; Annino, G. Commercial Vision Sensors and AI-Based Pose Estimation Frameworks for Markerless Motion Analysis in Sports and Exercises: A Mini Review. *Front. Physiol.* **2025**, *16*, 1649330. [CrossRef]
50. Sant'Ana, J.; Kons, R.L.; Detanico, D.; Diefenthaeler, F. The Use of Mobile Solutions for Biomechanical Assessment in Combat Sports: A Narrative Review. *Proc. Inst. Mech. Eng. Part P J. Sports Eng. Technol.* **2023**, *239*, 813–829.
51. Zhang, D.C.; Highhouse, S.; Nye, C.D. Development and Validation of the General Risk Propensity Scale (GRiPS). *J. Behav. Decis. Mak.* **2019**, *32*, 152–167. [CrossRef]
52. Della Villa, F.; Massa, B.; Bortolami, A.; Nanni, G.; Olmo, J.; Buckthorpe, M. Injury Mechanisms and Situational Patterns of Severe Lower Limb Muscle Injuries in Male Professional Football (Soccer) Players: A Systematic Video Analysis Study on 103 Cases. *Br. J. Sports Med.* **2023**, *57*, 1550–1558. [CrossRef]
53. Campoli, F.; Caprioli, L.; Cariati, I.; Edriss, S.; Romagnoli, C.; Bonaiuto, V.; Annino, G.; Padua, E. A Functional Recovery Program for Femoroacetabular Impingement in Two Professional Tennis Players: Outcomes at Two-Year Follow-Up. *J. Funct. Morphol. Kinesiol.* **2025**, *10*, 309. [CrossRef] [PubMed]
54. Caprioli, L.; Campoli, F.; Romagnoli, C.; Cariati, I.; Edriss, S.; Padua, E.; Bonaiuto, V.; Annino, G. Three Reasons for Playing the Tennis Forehand in Square Stance. *J. Funct. Morphol. Kinesiol.* **2025**, *10*, 215. [CrossRef]
55. Martin, C.; Sorel, A.; Touzard, P.; Bideau, B.; Gaborit, R.; DeGroot, H.; Kulpa, R. Influence of the Forehand Stance on Knee Biomechanics: Implications for Potential Injury Risks in Tennis Players. *J. Sports Sci.* **2021**, *39*, 992–1000. [CrossRef] [PubMed]

 https://doi.org/10.3390/healthcare14040430

56. Arboix-Alió, J.; Buscà, B.; Trabal, G.; Sarmento, H.; Vaz, V.; Moreno-Galcerán, D. Relationship between Upper Limb Muscle Power and Shooting Velocity in Elite Male Youth Rink Hockey Players. *Appl. Sci.* **2024**, *14*, 9368. [CrossRef]
57. Jiang, X.; Song, Y.; Sun, D.; Rong, M.; Mao, L.; Fekete, G. Sports Related Injury Mechanism on Ice Hockey Skills: A System Review. *J. Med. Imaging Health Inform.* **2020**, *10*, 1149–1158. [CrossRef]

https://doi.org/10.3390/healthcare14040430

healthcare MDPI

Systematic Review

Physical and Physiological Consequences of Babywearing on the Babywearer: A Systematic Review

Yaiza Taboada-Iglesias [1,2], Andrés Domínguez-Estévez [3], Clara Rodríguez-Gude [2,4,*] and Águeda Gutiérrez-Sánchez [1,2]

1 Special Didactics Department, Faculty of Science Education and Sport, Universidade de Vigo, 36005 Pontevedra, Spain; yaitaboada@uvigo.es (Y.T.-I.); agyra@uvigo.gal (Á.G.-S.)
2 Education, Physical Activity and Health Research Group (Gies10-DE3), Galicia Sur Health Research Institute (IIS), Universidade de Vigo, 36005 Pontevedra, Spain
3 Graduate in Physical Activity and Sport Sciences, Universidade de Vigo, 36005 Pontevedra, Spain; dominguezandrez10@gmail.com
4 Functional Biology and Health Sciences Department, Faculty of Physiotherapy, Universidade de Vigo, 36005 Pontevedra, Spain
* Correspondence: clara.rodriguez.gude@uvigo.es

Abstract: Background/Objectives: Babywearing is a carrying system that ensures consistent contact and proper posture between the baby and carrying adult, in which there is no age or weight limit, and it is rarely inadvisable. Although babywearing has been growing in popularity and acclaim due to the comfort and emotional closeness between the carrier and baby, there are a number of physical and physiological consequences for the adult carrier when using an ergonomic babywearing device, such as muscular, postural, cardiorespiratory, and energy expenditure, and the perception of effort and pain. The objective is to explore the physical implications affecting the carrier, as well as the subjective perception of strain and pain. **Methods**: A systematic review was carried out including articles up to December 2023 in the Web of Science (WOS), Medline, and SportDiscus databases. Studies dealing with ergonomic babywearing and the physical implications of babywearing were included; systematic reviews or case studies were excluded. **Results**: After applying the inclusion and exclusion criteria, a total of 14 original articles were obtained for analysis. Methodological quality was rated using the Joanna Briggs Institute Critical Appraisal Checklist for Analytical Cross-Sectional Studies with scores between 3 and 8 points. All articles included valid and reliable information on exposure, outcome measures, and results. **Conclusions**: The studies reviewed cover different aspects, such as muscle activation and postural stability, as well as specific ergonomic design for particular groups. In general terms, it seems that the use of certain babywearing devices, especially back or front carry, seems to be the one that generates fewer physiological alterations in the carriers compared to carrying babies in arms or other positions.

Keywords: baby carrier; energy expenditure; ergonomic carrying; muscle activation; posture

1. Introduction

The use of babywearing devices is spreading in the population, so much so that it has gained popularity and has experienced a remarkable increase in recent years, being a beneficial practice due to the constant contact between the baby and carrying adult [1]. Furthermore, appropriate babywearing has the potential to consistently support infants' spines [2]. This carrying practice involves carrying the baby in an ergonomically designed baby carrier, in which the baby's weight is evenly distributed. Although babywearing has been growing in popularity and praise due to the comfort and emotional closeness between the carrier and baby, there are still some precise questions and doubts about the physical and physiological implications for both the baby and adult. Furthermore, there are certain aspects that pediatricians and health professionals should inform in a correct manner and encourage good practice, as it is often not known what the appropriate devices are, whether it is conducted safely or not, and what the benefits are [3].

Babywearing can also involve differentiated strain between different types and methods of carrying. In the study by Fista et al. [4], subjective strain perception was measured using the BORG scale, in which the babywearer used three different types of baby carriers (a soft structured carrier, a ring sling, and a traditional shawl). The data indicated that the mechanism that caused the most strain was the baby carrier with a ring on the left shoulder because the sling rings made of metal put pressure on the left shoulder. In addition, they found that it also affected other areas such as the neck, back, and trunk.

The physical load is an important consideration to take into account, as it generates different muscle activations in the babywearer. Certain baby carriers generate less activation in the spinal muscles compared to other situations and therefore generate less injurious strains [5]. Yuk et al. [6], using electromyography (EMG), observed that different muscle patterns are activated depending on the method of carrying.

Just as there are muscle specificities of different physical activities, the practice of babywearing affects the adult's posture and gait. According to Azaman et al. [7], the pelvis, head, and shoulder are affected by carrying. In addition, carrying in the arms increases the load-bearing knee abduction moment by 8.7% and the load-bearing knee extension moment by 16.7% [8].

Also, the technique and duration of carrying and the physical characteristics of the carrying adult can alter cardiorespiratory aspects, and the energy expenditure related to ergonomic carrying can affect endurance and the ability to perform other physical tasks during the day. There are differences in energy costs [9] and perceived effort [10] between carrying a baby in the arms versus carrying a baby in a carry system.

Furthermore, the occurrence of pain is an important issue to consider when deciding whether to babywear or not. In the study by Mannen et al. [11], pain perception was analyzed using the Visual Analogue Scale. The results indicated that carrying adults experience more pain when carrying babies than when babywearing devices are used. This seemed to be due to the fact that when babies are carried, the body is in an asymmetrical position, and there are more areas of swaying.

It is important to assess the impact of babywearing in order to take appropriate measures to improve physical fitness. The design of baby carriers and their technique of use should be studied to minimize the risk of injury due to poor posture or increased muscle fatigue from prolonged carrying.

From the above, it appears that babywearing offers numerous benefits to ensure a comfortable and safe experience for the adult and baby, but it also has physical implications that affect the babywearer, and knowing the alterations produced by this practice of carrying and care, it will be possible to design exercise programs adapted to these populations, focused on preventing injuries or improving the experience.

It is important to better understand the physical implications for the adult using babywearing devices in order to generate exercise programs that prevent possible alterations or injuries. In addition, it seems relevant to provide information to parents, carrying adults, health professionals, and product designers in order to promote safe and healthy babywearing practices that benefit both the baby and the carrying adult.

Therefore, the aim of this paper is to explore the physical implications affecting the babywearer, focusing on physical and physiological aspects such as muscle activity, posture, and gait, and cardiorespiratory and energetic factors, as well as subjective perception of effort and pain.

2. Materials and Methods

2.1. Databases and Searches

This systematic review aimed to answer the following: What are the effects of different babywearing methods on (a) muscle activation, (b) postural stability, (c) energy expenditure, and (d) subjective pain and fatigue in healthy adults?

The PRISMA 2020 statement (Preferred Reporting Items for Systematic reviews and MetaAnalyses) [12] was followed for the search of the articles included in this review. This review protocol was developed prior to data extraction and is publicly available at OSF: https://osf.io/qjp4r/ (accessed on 29 December 2023). The search was conducted in the following databases: Web of Science (WOS), Medline, and SportDiscus, including results up to December 2023.

The following PICO(S) strategy was followed: Patient (babywearers); intervention (physical and physiological implications); comparison (other carrying methods); outcome (effects of babywearing).

The search strategy was applied independently in each database following the particularities of each one. The Medical Subject Heading (MESH) terms used in the search were "Physical fitness" [Mesh], "Postural Balance" [Mesh] and "Biomechanical phenomena" [Mesh]. In addition, the keywords used to identify articles on the subject of this review were 'baby carrier', 'ergonomic carrier', 'babywearing', 'baby carrying', combined with 'electromyography', 'muscle activity', 'postural stability', 'body balance', 'ergonomic', 'center of pressure', 'physical condition', and 'posture'. The Boolean operators OR and AND were used to link the terms and establish the search equations (Table 1).

Table 1. Search equations from different databases.

DB	Search Equation
MEDLINE	("baby carrier" OR "ergonomic carrier" OR "Baby carrying" OR "Babywearing") AND ("muscle activity" OR "electromyography" OR "postural stability" OR "Ergonomic" OR "center of pressure" OR "body balance" OR "physical condition" OR "Physical fitness" OR "Postural Balance" OR "Biomechanical phenomena" OR "Posture")
SPORTDISCUS	("baby carrier" OR "ergonomic carrier" OR "Baby carrying" OR "Babywearing") AND ("muscle activity" OR "electromyography" OR "postural stability" OR "Ergonomic" OR "center of pressure" OR "body balance" OR "physical condition" OR "Physical fitness" OR "Postural Balance" OR "Biomechanical phenomena" OR "Posture")
WEB OF SCIENCE	(((ALL = (baby carrier)) OR ALL = (ergonomic carrier)) OR ALL = (baby carrying)) AND ((((((((((ALL = (muscle activity)) OR ALL = (electromyography)) OR ALL = (postural stability)) OR ALL = (ergonomic)) OR ALL = (center of pressure)) OR ALL = (body balance)) OR ALL = (physical condition)) OR ALL = (physical fitness)) OR ALL = (Postural Balance)) OR ALL = (biomechanical phenomena)) OR ALL = (posture))

DB: databases.

All studies were assessed independently by two reviewers. Each reviewer screened titles and abstracts to obtain relevant full articles which were assessed against the inclusion and exclusion criteria described. In case of a lack of consensus, the judgment of a third reviewer prevailed.

2.2. Selection of Studies and Selection Criteria

For the selection of articles, studies dealing with babywearing and the physical implications of babywearing were set as inclusion criteria. Exclusion criteria were systematic reviews or case studies (Table 2).

Table 2. Inclusion and exclusion criteria.

Inclusion Criteria	Exclusion Criteria
- Studies dealing with babywearing - Physical or physiological implications for the adult carrying the baby (muscular voluntary contraction, center of pressure, heart rate, visual analogue scale, etc.).	- Systematic reviews - Case studies

The search identified 223 articles in the three databases, of which 9 were eliminated as duplicates. Of the 17 full-text articles assessed, 10 were excluded due to the fact that they were case studies, reviews, or articles that did not address the topic, resulting in 7 studies from the database search. Notably, 7 additional studies were identified through citation searching, yielding a total of 14 studies for inclusion. The entire process detailing the study selection steps can be found in the PRISMA flowchart (Figure 1).

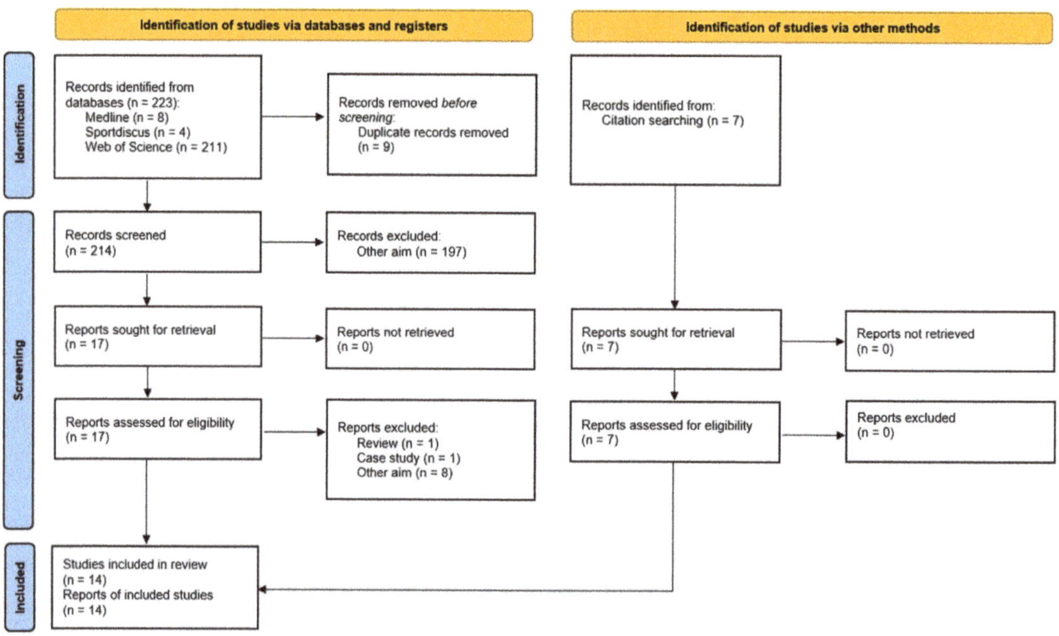

Figure 1. PRISMA flowchart of the item selection process.

2.3. Variables

This research includes data on the effects of babywearing on the babywearer's body, including variables such as muscle activation, load distribution and pressure, skin temperature, heart rate, stability, posture, balance, pain, gait kinematics, volumes, and respiratory rate, among others. For the interpretation of the results, results with statistical significance were compared. When studies use different units of measurement, results shall be standardized as far as possible. In addition, if the results provided are by subgroups, these shall be taken into account in the analysis.

2.4. Assessment of Methodological Quality and Risk of Bias of Individual Studies

The Joanna Briggs Institute Critical Appraisal Checklist for Analytical Cross-Sectional Studies (JBI) scale for analytical cross-sectional studies was used for the analysis of methodological quality [13].

The JBI scale uses eight criteria to assess the overall methodological quality of a study. Criteria for inclusion: sample inclusion criteria; description of subjects and settings; valid and reliable exposure measure; objective and standard measure of condition; identification of confounders; strategies to address confounders; valid and reliable outcome measure; and adequate statistical analysis. The final score ranges from 0 to 8 points. There is no ranking criterion for study quality. For ease of interpretation, we classified the methodological quality score, regardless of the scale used, as low (0–3 points), medium (4–6 points), and high (>6 points), as was conducted in a previous study [14].

3. Results

Methodological quality analysis yielded scores ranging from 3 to 8 points. One article scored low [15], nine scored medium [4–9,16–18], and four scored high [11,19–21] (Table 3). All studies met criteria 3 (exposure was measured in a valid and reliable manner), 4 (objective and standardized criteria were used to measure the condition), and 7 (outcomes were measured in a valid and reliable manner).

Table 3. Methodological quality scores of the "Joanna Briggs Institute Critical Appraisal Checklist for Analytical Cross-Sectional Studies".

Author (Year of Publication)	1	2	3	4	5	6	7	8	Score *
Wu et al. (2017) [21]	+	+	+	+	−	+	+	+	7
Chen et al. (2019) [16]	−	+	+	+	−	+	+	+	6
Azaman et al. (2017) [7]	+	+	+	+	−	−	+	+	6
Lee & Hong (2018) [18]	+	−	+	+	−	−	+	+	5
Wall-Scheffler et al. (2007) [9]	−	+	+	+	−	−	+	−	5
Havens et al. (2020) [17]	+	+	+	+	−	−	+	+	6
Ohashi et al. (2018) [20]	+	−	+	+	+	+	+	+	7
Mannen et al. (2020) [11]	+	+	+	+	+	+	+	+	8
Fista et al. (2019) [4]	−	+	+	+	−	−	+	−	4
Williams et al. (2019) [8]	+	+	+	+	−	−	+	+	6
Yuk et al. (2010) [6]	+	+	+	+	−	−	+	+	6
Hyun & Ryew (2018) [19]	−	+	+	+	+	+	+	+	7
Fagundes et al. (2016) [5]	+	+	+	+	−	−	+	+	6
Atthawuttikul & Khongkharat (2021) [15]	−	−	+	+	−	−	+	−	3

1. Were the criteria for inclusion in the sample clearly defined? 2. Were the study subjects and the setting described in detail? 3. Was the exposure measured in a valid and reliable way? 4. Were objective, standard criteria used for measurement of the condition? 5. Were confounding factors identified? 6. Were strategies to deal with confounding factors stated? 7. Were the outcomes measured in a valid and reliable way? 8. Was appropriate statistical analysis used? +: Yes; −: No. * The colors represent the different scores: red for low (0–3 points), orange for medium (4–6 points), and green for high (>6 points).

Table 4 showed the different types of carrying evaluated in each of the studies, while Table 5 summarized the main results and research characteristics of the studies included in this review, grouped by the different variables studied. We found that variables such as muscle activation have been evaluated in four studies [5,6,18,21]. Posture or stability has been investigated in six of the studies [4,7–9,15,17], while foot pressure or center of pressure has been investigated in five [6,7,11,18,19]. Physiological variables such as heart rate, skin temperature, or respiratory values have been evaluated in four of the studies [4,16,20,21].

Table 4. Types of carrying evaluated in each of the included studies.

	Load Type	**Frontal Load**		**Back Load**		**Side Load**	**Carry**	**No**	**Figure**
	(kg)	Backpack	Sling	Backpack	Sling	Sling	in arms	load	included
Wu et al. (2017) [21]	D (7 & 10)	X *	X						X
Chen et al. (2019) [16]	D (up to 7)	X *		X *					X
Azaman et al. (2017) [7]	D (5)		X		X	X	X	X	X
Lee & Hong (2018) [18]	D (7.6)	X *							X
Wall-Scheffler et al. (2007) [9]	D (7.6)				X		X		
Havens et al. (2020) [17]	D (5)	X					X	X	X
Ohashi et al. (2018) [20]	D (8.4)	X		X					X
Mannen et al. (2020) [11]	D (6 m)	X					X	X	X
Fista et al. (2019) [4]	D (7.3)	X	X *						X
Williams et al. (2019) [8]	D (2.7)	X					X	X	X
Yuk et al. (2010) [6]	D (7.6)	X	X	X				X	X
Hyun & Ryew (2018) [19]	B (<1 y, mean 10.9)			X				X	X
Fagundes et al. (2016) [5]	D (6)	X	X				X	X	X
Atthawuttikul & Khongkharat (2021) [15]	S	X *							X

* Indicates that the same study evaluated different baby carriers within the same type of load or subvariations within the same carrying device (e.g., tight vs. loose fit); B: baby; D: dummy; m: months; S: load simulated with software; y: year old; X: indicates the types of carrying included in each investigation.

Table 5. Summary of studies included in the review.

Author (Year)	**Sample**	**Scope/Variables Analyzed**	**Intervention/Methods**	**Results**
Fagundes et al. (2016) [5]	N = 20 ♀ healthy right-handed women without previous births (23.4 ± 1.39 years)	-Program EMG Lab V1.1. (lower trapezius and lumbar spinal erectors)	-The women walked for 3 min without load at a speed of 6 km/h. -In each baby-carrying situation, data were recorded for 60 s. -Collections were performed: (A) With the baby in a horizontal position, with the head facing the right side. (B) With the baby on your lap in an upright position. (C) Using kangaroo baby carrier, with arms alongside the body. (D) Using a sling (hammock) with the volunteer's arms alongside the body. (E) No load (Control).	EMG in -Load shape [$F_{(4, 59)} = 17.1$ $p < 0.001$] and side [$F_{(1, 59)} = 89.6$ $p < 0.001$] affected the intensity of erector spinae muscle activity. -Load shape [$F_{(4, 59)} = 6.4$ $p < 0.001$] and side [$F_{(1, 59)} = 59.9$ $p < 0.001$] affected the intensity of trapezius muscle descending fiber activity. -The trapezius obtained greater activation ($p < 0.001$) in form (a) than in forms (b), (c), and (e). -The left side, in all forms of loading, had the same intensity of activation of the trapezius muscle. -On the right side, form (a) showed greater activation than forms (e), (d), and (b). -EMG activity in the erector spinae muscle in form (b) was higher than in forms (a), (c), and (e). -Carrying form (d) showed greater activation than forms (c) and (e). The kangaroo carrier form generated less activation in the spinal muscles compared to other situations.
Yuk et al. (2010) [6]	N = 31 ♀ (23.2 ± 2.39 years)	-EMG (internal oblique, T4, L3, and L5 paravertebral, vastus medialis, biceps femoris, tibialis anterior, and gastrocnemius). -MATSacnSystem pressure foot platform.	Standing in all 4 positions: (A) Standing without load (SWC) (B) Carrying in front (LBC-F) (C) Carrying behind (LBC-B) (D) In shoulder carry (SC)	EMG: -Significant differences were found in the activation of biceps femoris (higher in LCB-F and lower in LCB-B), T4 (higher in LCB-F and LCB-B), L3 (higher in LCB-F, lower in LCB-B), L5 (higher in LCB-F, lower in LCB-B), and paravertebral ($p < 0.05$). -The other muscles did not show significant differences Foot pressure platform: -The pressure platform in the three forms of carrying obtained significant differences in the medial area of the right foot with respect to SWC.

Table 5. *Cont.*

Author (Year)	Sample	Scope/Variables Analyzed	Intervention/Methods	Results
Wu et al. (2017) [21]	N = 10 women (27.6 ± 3.8) and 10 men (27.8 ± 4.5)	-EMG (right side muscles: upper trapezius, rectus abdominis, erector spinae). -Skin temp. (upper back: midpoint between C7 and acromion; abdomen: 3 cm above the umbilicus). Shoulder pressure distribution. Heart rate.	The intervention was carried out on two different days. There were 6 combinations (3 types of baby carriers and 2 weights). In each combination, the baby was carried walking at a comfortable speed for 20 min while moving the arms freely. A 10 min break was taken between each combination.	EMG: -Upper trapezius and upper erector spinae in males ($p < 0.001$, $p = 0.047$, respectively), and rectus abdominis was significantly greater in females ($p < 0.001$). -Baby weight: upper trapezius and erector spinae were significantly greater when carrying a 10 kg baby than when carrying a 7 kg baby ($p < 0.001$). -Upper trapezius was significantly affected by baby carrier type: lower when using baby carrier type A than when using baby carrier type B, while baby carrier type C produced a similar response to the other two carriers. Body skin temperature: -Abdominal skin temp was higher in females ($p < 0.05$). -Carrier effect: Upper back temp was significantly different among the three carriers ($p < 0.001$). Type B produced the highest upper back skin temperature, while the use of type A and C carriers produced a lower upper back skin temperature. -Effect of weight: carrying a 7 kg baby resulted in higher abdominal skin temp ($p < 0.001$). Shoulder pressure distribution: -Significant differences according to baby carrier in shoulder pressure ($p < 0.05$) and maximum shoulder pressure ($p < 0.001$): type A produced the highest shoulder pressure and the highest maximum shoulder pressure, while baby carrier types B and C produced lower shoulder pressure, and baby carrier type B produced the lowest maximum shoulder pressure. Baby weight: the heavier the baby, the greater the pressure and the greater the maximum shoulder pressure. Heart rate: -Mean HR was higher in females ($p < 0.05$). -Baby weight: exercise intensity was greater with a 10 kg baby ($p < 0.05$).
Lee & Hong (2018) [18]	Healthy ♀ between 26 and 39 years	-COP: Foot pressure -Stability, comfort, and subjective fatigue -EMG: % of MVC	The following variables were measured using 3 types of baby carriers (X-type, H-type, and H-hip-type) and in two positions (fitted and loose). At rest and after walking for 30 min (with 30 min rest between carrier types). -COP: Body pressure measuring device (60 frames/s for 2 min). -EMG: Neck extensors, lower trapezius, thoracic and lumbar spinal erectors, rectus femoris, biceps femoris, tibialis anterior, medial calf. -Stability, comfort (shoulders, chest, and waist), and subjective fatigue: After 30 min walking (11-point Likert scale and Borg's CR-10 scale).	Stability: -The babywearers showed differences in medial/lateral shifts ($p < 0.05$), and the babywearing devices showed significant antero/posterior and diagonal differences ($p < 0.05$). -Antero/posterior displacement was greater in the H-type than in the H-hip type, with the H-type showing less stability than the other two. -Changes in COP, COP displacement, COP velocity, and anterior/posterior movement increased when baby carriers were used loosely compared to when they were used tightly ($p < 0.01$). Muscle fatigue: -Carrying types and mode only had significant interaction with fatigue in the medial gastrocnemius ($p < 0.01$). -Among the baby carrier types, X-type generated more muscle fatigue in the lower trapezius, thoracic spinal erectors, and biceps femoris than the other types. -The manner of use also resulted in differences in muscle fatigue. Subjective fatigue: -The center of mass shifted downwards when the carriers were worn loose, increasing pressure on the waist and femoral region. Comfort: -At the shoulders, it is more satisfactory when baby carriers are worn snug ($p < 0.01$), but comfort at the chest is better when loose ($p < 0.01$). -Waist comfort is better in the X-type ($p < 0.01$). They conclude that subjective wearing comfort worsens the more the body is covered, wrapped, and pressed, regardless of postural stability or muscle fatigue.
Azaman et al. (2017) [7]	N = 15 healthy ♀ (23.1 ± 1.03 years)	-COP: Distribution of M and Force in x, y, z axes. -Posture: Joint displacement (3D ROM of the markers located at the head, shoulders, pelvis, hip, knee, and ankle).	-All participants were measured under the following conditions: (A) No load (control) (B) Loaded (L) (C) Loaded with baby carrier in front (LBC-F) (D) Loaded with baby carrier on the side (LBC-S) (F) Loaded with baby carrier on the back (LBC-B) -They stood for 1 min on the platform and rested for 5 min between postures.	COP: -Anterior displacement in L and LBC-F relative to control ($p < 0.05$). -LBC-F appears to displace the COP less than without baby carrier, but not significantly so. -LBC-F produces less anterior-posterior displacement and more lateral displacement than LBC-S or LBC-B but not significant ($p > 0.05$). Posture: -Pelvis, head, and shoulder are affected by load. -LBC-F produces less anteroposterior deviation of the joints than the other baby carrier situations.
Williams et al. (2019) [8]	N = 18 healthy ♀ (22.67 ± 2.08 years)	-Posture: camera and reflective markers	-3 walking sessions under the following conditions: (A) A baseline of three minutes unloaded (UL). (B) 15 min while carrying an infant dummy (2.73 kg) in arms (IA) (C) 15 min while babywearing an infant dummy in a structured baby carrier in an anterior position (BC)	-IA: increases the mechanical load on the knee and hip joints in the frontal plane by increasing joint moments. Arm carry increases the loading knee abduction moment by 8.7% and the loading knee extension moment by 16.7%. -BC: more similar to unloaded gait. -They conclude that during prolonged transport, babywearers may choose to use a baby carrier instead of carrying the baby in their arms.
Hyun & Ryew. (2018) [19]	N = 9 ♀ experienced in baby delivering (27.88 ± 2.71 years)	-1st and 2nd peak vertical force (PVF) -Medial-lateral and anteroposterior COPs -Extrapolated center of mass (XCoM). -Leg stiffness.	-GRF system and camera (4 units). -All participants wore 6 cm high heels. Randomly: (A) In normal conditions (no load). (B) Babywearing using a rear baby carrier.	-1st PVF: statistically significant differences according to the use of high heels and walking conditions, being higher when carrying a baby. -2nd PVF: statistically significant differences according to walking conditions. -Medial-lateral COP: showed statistically significant differences according to heel height and walking conditions. -Anteroposterior COP: showed no statistically significant differences according to heel shoe use and walking conditions during gait. -XCoM: showed statistically significant differences in the case of wearing heels. -Leg stiffness: showed statistically significant differences in the case of wearing heeled shoes and walking conditions.
Fista et al. (2019) [4]	N = 12 ♀ (between 20 and 22 years)	Posture (horizontal cranial, cranio-vertebral, and sagittal angles). -HR. -Borg discomfort (shoulders, neck, back, and trunk). -ABC scale (balance, self-confidence not to lose balance).	-Walking on a treadmill for 10 min. 3 different types of baby carriers: (A) SSC harness (B) Jarík (C) Ring sling	Posture: -All types of baby carriers produced a mean value of 49–52° in the sagittal angle. -In the horizontal cranial angle, the SSC-type sling provided the best change in posture. ABC scale: -According to the results of the ABC scale questionnaire, the SSC sling provided a higher level of confidence than the Jarík and the ring sling. Pain: The ring sling and the Jarík produced more pain in the left shoulder than the SSC sling.

Table 5. *Cont.*

Author (Year)	Sample	Scope/Variables Analyzed	Intervention/Methods	Results
Mannen et al. (2020) [11]	N = 10 ♀ healthy nulliparous (27.4 ± 4.1 years)	-Pain: VAS -COP: 2 × 40 × 40 cm force plates during testing at 1000 Hz.	Stand still for 15 min on a force platform (COP) and VAS after exposure in each of the following conditions: (A) No load (B) Carrying a dummy in arms (C) Babywearing a dummy	Pain: -30% reported pain during unloading and carrying -50% reported pain when carrying in arms COP -Participants shifted their weight more frequently, spent more time in an asymmetrical position, and had greater areas of swinging in arm carry. -In the comparison between pain and non-pain sufferers, pain sufferers remained more stationary in all conditions; although the baby carrier caused pain participants to shift their weight more often, this was a positive change.
Havens et al. (2020) [17]	N = 10 ♀ healthy nulliparous (27.4 ± 4.1 years)	-Motion capture based on movements -Force platform. -Kinematics: (step length, step time, support time, gait speed, and step width). -GRF	Assess how they walk and bend down to pick up an object: (A) Without weight (B) In arms (C) Carrying in a baby carrier	Gait: -Carrying in arms: greater vertical GRF and momentum, and braking force compared to non-weight bearing. Greater back extension. -Significant but small differences (<5°) between conditions were found in lower limb kinematics. -2.2% greater stride length in 'weightless' compared to 'in arms'. Recovery: -The majority of individuals performed the squat technique to retrieve the object. -There were significant differences in lower limb kinematics at squat depth between right and left legs. There were no differences in timing between the downward and upward phases of the squat between conditions.
Wall-Scheffler et al. (2007) [9]	N = 6 ♀ of reproductive age (20.5 ± 0.8 years)	-VO2max -Anthropometry: Lower limbs, mass, and height. -Kinematics: Stride length and contact time	-4 sessions of treadmill walking of 15 min: (A) Control: weight on waist. (B) Control 2: weight on belt and no braking. (C) Carrying dummy in arms (D) Carrying the baby carrier dummy in anterior position	Anthropometry: -Bitrochanteric width correlates significantly with stride length and contact time under the most normal level. Energy cost: -Significant differences between A and B; B and C; A and C; C and D. Most interestingly, the average increase in cost of carrying a baby in arms versus babywearing in a sling is 16% (ranging from 13% to 25% increase). Kinematics: -Normalized stride lengths are shorter during carrying in arms than during the other experimental conditions.
Ohashi et al. (2018) [20]	N = 14 healthy young adults	-Heart rate (HR) -Oxygen uptake (V4 O2) -Ventilation/minute (V4 E) -Tidal volume (TV) -Respiratory exchange rate (R) -Respiratory rate (RR) -Last-minute values for each degree were averaged.	-Individualized walking speed at 30% of maximum oxygen uptake at 0% grade incline. -The test started at 0% grade walking on the treadmill and increased by 2% every 5 min up to 8%. The test was performed in a randomized fashion: (A) Front condition (F) (infant forward facing with lullaby belt). (B) Back condition (B) (infant backwards with lullaby belt).	-HR, V4 O2, V4 E, TV, R, and RR increased significantly with increasing grade in each condition (every 5 min). -There were no significant differences in interaction effects in HR, V4 O2, V4 E, TV, R, and RR. -No significant differences were found in the interactions between obliquity, condition, and sex for any of the items.
Chen et al. (2019) [16]	N = 10 ♀ and 10 males (24.0 ± 2.5)	-MAWC -%HR = (HR work − HR rest) × 100% -Perceived exertion (Borg's CR-10 scale) in the whole body, neck, right shoulder, left shoulder, upper back, middle back, lower back, and abdomen	Eight transport tasks were performed. HR and MAWC were measured during each task. At the completion of each task, the Borg CR-10 was run. Type of carrier: (A) Padded shoulder straps and belt, with waist and abdomen support. (B) Two-part backpack, which distributes the weight. Carrying time: 1 h and 4 h Type of carrying: front and back	MAWC, obtained $p < 0.05$ in: -Sex: males (16.9 kg) vs. females (13.2 kg). -Rear carry (15.4 kg) vs. front carry (14.7 kg). -Type of carry: A = 15.6 kg vs. A = 14.5 kg. -Time: 1 h (16.2 kg) vs. 4 h (11.7 kg). %FC: carrying 1 h (19.3%) vs. 4 h (14.6%). $p < 0.01$ Perceived effort -Whole body: $p < 0.05$ in time (4.6 in 1 h vs. 4.0 in 4 h). -Mid back: $p < 0.05$ being higher in women (3.2) than in men (2.3). -Lower back: women (4.7) higher than men (3.5) ($p < 0.01$); front carrying (4.5) higher than back carrying (3.6) ($p < 0.01$); 1 h carrying (4.5) higher than 4 h carrying (3.6) ($p < 0.01$) and type A (4.5) higher than type B (3.7) ($p < 0.05$).
Atthawuttikul & Khongkharat (2021) [15]	Older people	-Questionnaire -Maximum load/transporter.	-The three 3D models were imported into force simulation software along with Earth gravity constant = ~9600 Nm/s. Stiffness = ~0.40 MPa. Flexibility = ~0.26 MPa. Durability = ~1.6 MPa. against impact force.	-Model D3 was able to withstand the highest load. -Model D1 supported the lowest load. -The four main factors in the ergonomic design for older people were the following: (1) the posture of their shoulders and hips while using the carrier. (2) the seat and backrest areas as load points of the baby carrier. (3) the load points on their body. (4) the type of baby carrier.

ABC Scale: Activities-Specific Balanced Confidence Scale; BC: baby carrying; cm: centimeters; COP: center of pressure; GRF: ground reaction force; h: hour; HR: heart rate; Hz: hertz; IA: in arms; kg: kilograms; km: kilometers; L: loaded; LBC-B: Loaded with baby carrier on the back; LBC-F: Loaded with baby carrier in front; LBC-S: Loaded with baby carrier on the side; M: Moment of the force plate; min: minutes; MAWC: maximum acceptable weight of carrying; MPa: megapascals; MVC: maximum voluntary contraction; Nm/s: newton per meter/second; R: Respiratory exchange rate; RR: respiratory rate; SC: shoulder carry; SSC: Soft Structured Carrier; SWC: Standing without load; Temp: temperature; TV: tidal volume; UL: unloaded; V4 E: ventilation/minute; V4 O2: oxygen uptake; VAS: visual analogue scale; VO2max: Maximum Oxygen Consumption; XCoM: Extrapolated center of mass; ♀: female.

4. Discussion

This paper has analyzed the physical and physiological consequences of babywearing on the babywearer. To the authors' knowledge, this is the first systematic review on this topic. The results analyzed in this review come from articles with acceptable methodological quality, with only one article rated with a low score on the JBI scale.

When interpreting the different results obtained in the studies, methodological differences have been observed, such as the use of dummies versus babies, the different walking or standing protocols used, as well as the different designs of carrying systems used, among others. Such heterogeneity in the studies has made direct comparability between them difficult.

4.1. Muscle Activity

Different types of baby carriers affect the muscle activation of the babywearer and in this case, EMG is a widely used tool. In the study by Fagundes et al. [5], an electromyographic analysis of the spinal muscles was performed during walking and with different baby carriers. In terms of the results, baby carriers that do not distribute the weight evenly generate more activation of the spinal muscles. In contrast, the kangaroo method activates these muscles the least compared to other situations. In the study by Yuk et al. [6], they also used EMG to study the activation of trunk and lower limb muscles such as the biceps femoris. Their results show that front babywearing (LBC-F) generates greater activation in all the muscles analyzed than back babywearing (LBC-B), which could result in greater muscle fatigue and injury with prolonged use. On the other hand, in a high-quality study [21], the activation of the upper trapezius was greater when carrying a two-part front-facing backpack than with a front-facing backpack with shoulder straps. In addition, upper trapezius and erector spinae activation was statistically significantly higher in males and also in heavier babies, while rectus abdominis activation was higher in females. Based on this, an ergonomic design that minimizes muscle loading and favors adequate weight distribution of the baby is important.

4.2. Posture and Gait

The use of baby carriers has a significant impact on the babywearer's posture and gait. Azaman et al. [7] found that baby carriers can alter the wearer's posture, increasing postural sway. Thus, according to the results analyzed, the pelvis, head, and trunk are affected by the load. Another curious fact is that carrying a baby carrier in the front produces less anteroposterior deviation of the joints than back or side baby carriers.

Along the same lines, Havens et al. [17] analyze how different methods of carrying the baby affect the carrier's posture during walking and picking up objects. Thus, carrying the baby with unequal weight and asymmetrical posture results in back extension, which affects the efficiency of movement. In terms of retrieval, most individuals performed the squat technique to retrieve the object from the floor, both while carrying it and with it in their arms.

And for its relationship with lower and upper limbs, the study by Williams et al. [8] also examines the babywearer's posture using different infant carrier methods, and the resulting data are similar to the previous study in that carrying in arms increases the carrying knee abduction moment by 8.7% and the carrying knee extension moment by 16.7%. Hyun and Ryew [19] studied the effects of carrying an infant using a rear carrier during high-heeled walking in high-quality research. After analyzing the 1st and 2nd peak vertical force (PVF), there are statistically significant differences according to the use of high heels and walking conditions. On the other hand, medial-lateral center of pressure (COP) and leg stiffness showed statistically significant differences according to heel height and walking conditions. This finding is particularly relevant for babywearers performing activities where posture and stability are crucial, such as walking on inclined or uneven surfaces.

4.3. Load

Another factor to consider is the weight of the baby. Chen et al. [16] investigated the maximum acceptable load during babywearing, finding that men carried more weight than women, that more weight could be carried in 1 h than in 4 h, that when back babywearing, the acceptable weight was greater than when front carrying, and that backpacks with shoulder straps carried more weight than two-part backpacks. These data will be important for babywearers to consider, as depending on the weight of the baby, the choice of both baby carrier and carrying position may vary. In addition, the length of use should also be considered, as excessive use can be harmful even with regard to the recommended weight for each device.

4.4. Cardiorespiratory Effects

The impact of baby carrier use on cardiorespiratory response and energy expenditure is another important determinant to consider. When assessing heart rate (HR), Wu et al. [21] found, in their high-quality study, that HR was statistically higher in women, and that the weight of the baby also affected exercise intensity, as it was higher when carrying a 10 kg baby than a 7 kg baby. Chen et al. [16] also assessed HR, finding that the percentage of maximum heart rate (%HR) was higher when carrying for 1 h than for 4 h. A study evaluating the relationship between the HR of babywearers and babies during babywearing also found that babywearing increases the babywearer's HR, but the baby's HR decreases, especially when the mother is carrying the baby [22].

In the high-quality study by Ohashi et al. [20], the respiratory response during downhill walking was analyzed by front and back carrying with baby carriers, and in both situations, the respiratory effort increased significantly. This effort is accompanied by higher energy expenditure, which leads to lower locomotion efficiency and greater fatigue during prolonged use. From a different perspective, the study by Wall-Scheffler et al. [9] analyzed the effects on the musculoskeletal system of carrying a baby using different carrying mechanisms. The results indicated that there is an average increase in the perceived physical effort when carrying a baby in arms compared to carrying a baby in a sling (16%, ranging from a 13% to a 25% increase). In addition, standardized stride lengths are shorter during carriage in arms than when using a front carrier. Following these explorations, it is of vital importance to design babywearing devices that promote ergonomic posture, reduce energy expenditure, and improve movement efficiency.

4.5. Fatigue and Pain

To assess comfort and fatigue during babywearing, perceived exertion can help us, even though it is a subjective measure. In the study by Chen et al. [16], front carrying had a higher value in perceived exertion compared to back carrying, both in the lower back and abdomen, as measured by the Borg CR-10 scale. Fista et al. [4] used a physiological and biomechanical approach to evaluate different methods of use (Soft Structured Carrier (SSC) harness, Jarik, and ring sling) of baby carriers. The data indicated that the mechanism that caused the most strain was the ring sling and the Jarik, especially on the left shoulder. The SSC-type harness provided the best change of posture and the highest level of confidence. Similarly, Lee and Hong [18] measured muscle fatigue and COP in different types of baby carriers. They found that designs that allow a more natural posture and distribute weight evenly reduce muscle fatigue. This reduction in muscle fatigue translates into less perceived strain on the part of the carrier, which is crucial for carrier acceptance and prolonged use, since the time spent carrying babies is considerable [23].

As with the previous variable, pain perception is also important to take into account when carrying and is a good indicator of whether the ergonomic design is adequate or not. To this end, the study by Mannen et al. [11], considered to be of good quality, investigated how different methods of carrying the baby (unloaded, carrying a dummy in arms, carrying a dummy) affect postural sway and pain during prolonged standing. The results indicated that 30% of the participants reported pain during unloading and carrying, while 50% reported pain during carrying. Participants shifted their weight more frequently as they spent more time in an asymmetrical position and had greater areas of swinging in weight bearing and therefore increased the perception of pain, especially in the lumbar region. In relation to the previous article and the pain that can be suffered in the back while carrying, one study [15], which had moderate methodological quality, suggested the need to design baby carriers that provide good lumbar support and distribute the weight in a balanced way, especially for older people, as this can reduce pain in the back and joints. Another factor pointed out by these authors is the posture of the shoulders and hips while using the baby carrier by the users.

4.6. Limitations, Future Lines of Research, and Practical Implications

In terms of limitations, while the chosen databases are major sources, a broader search might have captured additional relevant literature. The review includes studies with different experimental designs and measurement methods, which may limit the comparability of results. On the other hand, most of the studies focus on young and middle-aged adults, and most of them are conducted only on women, which makes it difficult to extrapolate results to the male or older population; however, the profile found in the studies corresponds to the population that tends to use these parenting aids the most. Furthermore, the interpretation of some of the variables studied, such as heart rate or muscle activation, may imply a difference in results depending on the characteristics of the wearer, including age, sex, and anthropometry. A number of studies are conducted in controlled settings and with dummies simulating babies rather than real children, which may not reflect the conditions of real, everyday use.

In terms of future lines of research, the long-term effects of baby carrier use on the health of the carriers in real, everyday conditions could be investigated, as well as extending studies to broader groups such as older people, individuals with disabilities, or different ethnicities. In addition, research can be conducted on the incorporation of new smart technologies in baby carrier design.

Furthermore, this information can serve as a basis for designers to improve the design of baby carriers, making them more ergonomic and adaptable to different carriers. As for health professionals, they should use this information to educate users about the best types of baby carriers and the importance of good posture. In addition, these experts should apply the knowledge to develop specific exercise and stretching programs for babywearers. As for parents, understanding the effects of different types of baby carriers helps them choose which one to use, given the wide variety available on the market.

5. Conclusions

The analysis carried out on the existing literature on the use of baby carriers and their relationship to carrier ergonomics reveals a number of important findings that should be considered by both health professionals and baby carrier designers. The studies under analysis cover different aspects, such as muscle activation and postural stability, as well as specific ergonomic design for particular groups. The synthesized evidence suggests that back carriers seem to be the least likely to cause physiological alterations in babywearers compared to babywearing babies in arms or other positions.

On the one hand, it has been shown that different ways of carrying the baby (front, back, or in arms) affect the electromyographic activity of the spinal muscles, and, in terms of muscle fatigue, it is essential that baby carriers minimize excessive activation of the trunk and lower limb muscles to reduce muscle fatigue and the risk of injury, as this can have a considerable impact on the user's musculoskeletal health in the long term, with kangaroo or back carry mode being found to generate the least activation.

On the other hand, depending on the type of baby carrier, these can influence the wearer's posture and gait, so a design that favors even weight distribution and supports a natural posture is crucial to maintain stability and gait efficiency.

Infant carrying methods also affect breathing and energy expenditure compared to carrying the baby in your arms, so the design should be optimized to reduce respiratory and energy expenditure, which can significantly improve the comfort and prolonged wearability of the baby carrier. Therefore, in addition to design factors and carrying modalities that minimize injury and improve the posture and stability of the carrier, intervention through physical exercise is important to reduce and prevent physical problems that may affect the carriers. It is also important to take into account the duration of use due to the load being carried, trying not to exceed the time limit, and taking breaks whenever possible to avoid injuries due to overexertion.

Author Contributions: Conceptualization, Y.T.-I.; methodology, Y.T.-I. and A.D.-E.; investigation, C.R.-G. and Á.G.-S.; resources, A.D.-E.; writing—original draft preparation, Y.T.-I. and A.D.-E.; writing—review and editing, Y.T.-I., C.R.-G., and Á.G.-S.; visualization, C.R.-G. and Á.G.-S.; supervision, Y.T.-I.; project administration, Y.T.-I. All authors have read and agreed to the published version of the manuscript.

Funding: This research received no external funding.

Institutional Review Board Statement: Not applicable.

Informed Consent Statement: Not applicable.

Data Availability Statement: No new data were created or analyzed in this study.

Conflicts of Interest: The authors declare no conflicts of interest.

Abbreviations

The following abbreviations are used in this manuscript:

EMG	Electromyography
PRISMA	Preferred Reporting Items for Systematic reviews and MetaAnalyses
WOS	Web of Science
PICO	Patient, Intervention, Comparison, Outcome
MESH	Medical Subject Heading
JBI	Joanna Briggs Institute Critical Appraisal Checklist for Analytical Cross-Sectional Studies
LBC-B	Loaded with baby carrier on the back
LBC-F	Loaded with baby carrier in front
PVF	Peak Vertical Force
COP	Center of pressure
HR	Heart Rate
SSC	Soft Structured Carrier

References

1. Williams, L.R.; Grisham, L.M.; Gebler-Wolfe, M.; Kelsch, K.; Bedrick, A.; Bader, M.Y. Nurse Perceptions of Babywearing for Neonates with Neonatal Abstinence Syndrome in the Neonatal Intensive Care Unit. *Adv. Neonatal. Care.* **2021**, *21*, 23–31. [CrossRef]
2. Siddicky, S.F.; Bumpass, D.B.; Krishnan, A.; Tackett, S.A.; McCarthy, R.E.; Mannen, E.M. Positioning and baby devices impact infant spinal muscle activity. *J. Biomech.* **2020**, *104*, 109741. [CrossRef]
3. López Acuña, E.S.; Salmerón Ruiz, M.A. El porteo ergonómico; Ergonomic babywearing. *Pediatr. Integral.* **2014**, *XVIII*, 774–780. (In Spanish)
4. Fista, B.; Widyanti, A.; Muslim, K.; Salma, S.A. Evaluation of Baby Carriers in Indonesia: Physiological and Biomechanical Approach. *IOP Conf. Ser. Mater. Sci. Eng.* **2019**, *598*, 012113. [CrossRef]

5. Fagundes, F.; Teixeira, F.; Camargo, L.; Mochizuki, L.; Amorim, C.; Soares, R. Análise eletromiográfica de músculos da coluna vertebral durante a marcha em diferentes formas de carregar o bebê; Electromyographic analysis of the spinal muscles during the gait in different ways to carry a baby. *Conscientiae Saúde* **2016**, *15*, 210–216. Available online: http://www.redalyc.org/articulo.oa?id=92949791005 (accessed on 29 December 2023). [CrossRef]
6. Yuk, G.C.; Park, R.J.; Lee, H.Y.; Lee, M.H.; Lee, J.H.; Kuk, J.S.; Jang, J.-S. The Effects of Baby Carrier and Sling in Muscle Activation of Trunk, Low Extremity and Foot Pressure. *J. Korean Soc. Phys. Med.* **2010**, *5*, 223–317.
7. Azaman, A.; Isa, N.M.; Dzahir, M.; Xiang, K.K. Effects of baby carrier on wearer's posture stability. *J. Mech. Eng.* **2017**, *SI 4*, 107–118. Available online: https://ir.uitm.edu.my/id/eprint/39240 (accessed on 29 December 2023).
8. Williams, L.; Standifird, T.; Madsen, M. Effects of infant transportation on lower extremity joint moments: Baby carrier versus carrying in-arms. *Gait Posture* **2019**, *70*, 168–174. [CrossRef] [PubMed]
9. Wall-Scheffler, C.; Geiger, K.; Steudel-Numbers, K. Infant carrying: The role of increased locomotory costs in early tool development. *Am. J. Phys. Anthropol.* **2007**, *133*, 841–846. [CrossRef]
10. Ojukwu, C.P.; Okafor, C.J.; Chukwu, S.C.; Anekwu, E.M.; Okemuo, A.J. Evaluation of selected cardiopulmonary and perceived exertion responses to four infant carrying methods utilised by African Mothers. *J. Obstet Gynaecol.* **2019**, *39*, 1098–1103. [CrossRef] [PubMed]
11. Mannen, E.; Havens, K.; Kahney, A.; Nelson-Wong, E. Baby-Carrying Method Impacts Caregiver Postural Sway and Pain During Prolonged Standing. *J. Womens Health* **2020**, *44*, 47–53. [CrossRef]
12. Page, M.J.; McKenzie, J.E.; Bossuyt, P.M.; Boutron, I.; Hoffmann, T.C.; Mulrow, C.D.; Shamseer, L.; Tetzlaff, J.M.; Akl, E.A.; Brennan, S.E.; et al. The PRISMA 2020 statement: An updated guideline for reporting systematic reviews. *BMJ* **2021**, *372*, n71. [CrossRef] [PubMed]
13. Joanna Briggs Institute. Checklist for Analytical Cross Sectional Studies Critical Appraisal. 2020. Available online: https://jbi.global/sites/default/files/2020-08/Checklist_for_Analytical_Cross_Sectional_Studies.pdf (accessed on 27 July 2022).
14. Leno-Durán, E.; Micha-Mabale, M.; García-Pérez, M.; Bueno-Cavanillas, A.; Barrios-Rodríguez, R.; Requena, P. Influencia de la dieta en el riesgo de infección y de gravedad de la COVID-19: Una revisión sistemática; Influence of diet in COVID-19 infection and severity risk: A systematic review. *Nutr. Hosp.* **2023**, *40*, 444–456. (In Spanish) [CrossRef] [PubMed]
15. Atthawuttikul, A.; Khongkharat, S. Factors in Ergonomic Design of 6-to-18-month Baby Carriers for Elderly People. *Pertanika J. Sci.* **2021**, *29*, 1097–1108. [CrossRef]
16. Chen, T.H.; Kao, Y.Y.; Wang, M.J.J. The Psychophysical Evaluations of Baby Carriers. In *Advances in Physical Ergonomics & Human Factors*; Goonetilleke, R.S., Karwowski, W., Eds.; Springer International Publishing: Cham, Switzerland, 2019; pp. 234–241.
17. Havens, K.L.; Severin, A.C.; Bumpass, D.B.; Mannen, E.M. Infant carrying method impacts caregiver posture and loading during gait and item retrieval. *Gait Posture* **2020**, *80*, 117–123. [CrossRef]
18. Lee, H.; Hong, K. Type and wearing method-dependent COP and muscle fatigue measurement of baby carriers for the development of smart baby carriers. *Int. J. Cloth. Sci. Technol.* **2018**, *30*, 610–627. [CrossRef]
19. Hyun, S.H.; Ryew, C.C. Effect of lower limb kinetic on carrying infant by hip seat carrier during high heel gait. *J. Exerc. Rehabil.* **2018**, *14*, 1092–1095. [CrossRef]
20. Ohashi, K.; Ono, K.; Kawate, Y.; Watase, R.; Ishikawa, A. Respiratory response during upslope walking with different ways to carry a baby using baby carrier. *Jpn. J. Phys. Fit. Sports Med.* **2018**, *67*, 303–309. (In Japanese) [CrossRef]
21. Wu, C.Y.; Huang, H.R.; Wang, M.J. Baby carriers: A comparison of traditional sling and front-worn, rear-facing harness carriers. *Ergonomics* **2017**, *60*, 111–117. [CrossRef]
22. Han, J.H.; Rankin, L.; Lee, H.; Feng, D.; Grisham, L.M.; Benfield, R. Infant and parent heart rates during a babywearing procedure: Evidence for autonomic coregulation. *Infant Behav. Dev.* **2024**, *77*, 101996. [CrossRef]
23. Nadeem, A.; Faisal, S.; Waqas, S. Association Between Infant Carrying Methods, Duration, And Trunk Position Among Nursing Mothers of Lahore. *J. Riphah. Coll. Rehabili. Sci.* **2024**, *12*, 213–218. [CrossRef]

healthcare

MDPI

Systematic Review

Effects of Exercise-Based Rehabilitation on Lumbar Degenerative Disc Disease: A Systematic Review

Shirin Aali [1], Farhad Rezazadeh [2], Fariborz Imani [2], Mahsa Nabati Sefidekhan [2], Georgian Badicu [3], Luca Poli [4,*], Francesco Fischetti [4,*], Stefania Cataldi [5,†] and Gianpiero Greco [4,†]

1 Department of Physical Education, Farhangian University, P.O. Box 889-14665, Tehran 19396-14464, Iran; sh.aali@cfu.ac.ir

2 Department of Sports Biomechanics, Faculty of Educational Sciences and Psychology, University of Mohaghegh Ardabili, Ardabil 56199-11367, Iran; rezazadeh.farhad@uma.ac.ir (F.R.); fariborzimani@uma.ac.ir (F.I.); mahsaaanabatiii@gmail.com (M.N.S.)

3 Department of Physical Education and Special Motricity, Faculty of Physical Education and Mountain Sports, Transilvania University of Braşov, 500068 Braşov, Romania; georgian.badicu@unitbv.ro

4 Department of Translational Biomedicine and Neuroscience (DiBraiN), University of Study of Bari, 70124 Bari, Italy; gianpiero.greco@uniba.it

5 Department of Education and Sport Sciences, Pegaso Telematic University, 80143 Naples, Italy; stefania.cataldi@unipegaso.it

* Correspondence: luca.poli@uniba.it (L.P.); francesco.fischetti@uniba.it (F.F.)

† These authors share the last authorship.

Abstract: Background: This systematic review evaluates the efficacy of rehabilitation-focused exercise interventions for lumbar degenerative disc disease (DDD), a leading cause of chronic low back pain. **Methods:** Following PRISMA guidelines, a comprehensive search was conducted across international and regional databases (PubMed, Scopus, Web of Science, Magiran, SID, and Noormags) covering the period from January 2010 to January 2025. The review protocol was registered with the International Prospective Register of Systematic Reviews (PROSPERO) under registration number CRD420251088811. Using keywords such as "lumbar DDD," "exercise therapy," and "rehabilitation," a total of 2495 records were identified. After screening, 20 studies—including clinical trials, quasi-experimental, and experimental designs—met the inclusion criteria and were assessed using the McMaster Critical Review Form for Quantitative Studies. **Results:** Interventions such as hydrotherapy, core stability training, Pilates, and suspension exercises were found to significantly reduce pain and improve functional outcomes. While multimodal approaches (e.g., aquatic exercise combined with acupuncture) showed positive effects, the comparative studies revealed no significant differences between modalities. Suspension training demonstrated superior efficacy in pain reduction compared to isolated core stability exercises. The methodological quality of included studies ranged from good to excellent, with the majority rated as very good or excellent (McMaster scores: 8 "excellent," 7 "very good," and 5 "good"). Common limitations among the studies included methodological heterogeneity, small sample sizes (n = 14–30), and insufficient long-term follow-up. **Conclusions:** Exercise-based rehabilitation is an effective strategy for managing lumbar DDD. Evidence particularly supports the use of suspension training and aquatic therapy for superior improvements in pain and functional outcomes. Future research should aim to adopt standardized protocols, recruit larger sample sizes, and include extended follow-up periods to produce more robust and generalizable findings.

Keywords: corrective exercises; lumbar DDD; therapeutic exercise; physical therapy

1. Introduction

Low back pain (LBP) is a multifactorial clinical syndrome characterized by pain, stiffness, or muscular tension localized between the lower rib margin and the gluteal folds, with or without radiating sciatic symptoms [1]. As the leading global cause of disability, LBP affected approximately 619 million people worldwide in 2020, with projections estimating an increase to 843 million by 2050, driven primarily by aging populations and increasingly sedentary lifestyles [1].

The World Health Organization's Global Burden of Disease Study consistently ranks LBP as the top contributor to years lived with disability (YLDs), exceeding the burden of all other musculoskeletal conditions combined [1,2]. The financial burden of LBP is considerable, accounting for 1–2% of the gross domestic product in developed countries through both direct costs (e.g., imaging, pharmacotherapy, surgery) and indirect costs (e.g., productivity loss, disability claims). In the United States alone, annual expenditures exceed $100 billion, with nearly two-thirds attributed to indirect workplace-related costs [3]. This economic burden disproportionately affects blue-collar workers and middle-aged adults, posing significant challenges for the labor force [2,3].

According to research findings, degenerative disc disease (DDD), encompassing intervertebral disc disorders, has a striking prevalence of 54% and is the leading cause of chronic back pain [4]. This prevalent neuromuscular disorder primarily affects the lumbar and cervical regions of the spine, typically presenting with a triad of debilitating symptoms: localized or radiating pain, muscle weakness, and restricted range of motion [4]. Among its multifactorial causes, persistent pain remains the primary contributor to both temporary and permanent occupational disability [4]. Supporting this, a comparative study by Radziszewski reported work productivity losses exceeding 40% among patients with chronic lumbar DDD. These findings collectively establish comprehensive pain management as a therapeutic cornerstone, which, when combined with functional restoration, serves as the primary indicator of successful treatment outcomes [5]. Extensive research indicates that 70–85% of individuals experience LBP at least once during their lifetime, a prevalence shaped by lifestyle, occupational demands, ageing, and genetic predisposition [6]. Among these cases, nearly 5% progress to disc herniation, in which intervertebral disc bulging becomes a primary source of pain and core muscle dysfunction [7,8]. Although the exact pathological mechanisms remain incompletely understood, several modifiable risk factors—particularly poor posture, inadequate seating ergonomics, and prolonged sedentary behavior—are known to accelerate both disc degeneration and atrophy of core stabilizing muscles [9,10]. These factors increase mechanical stress on intervertebral discs, leading to structural alterations and impaired disc metabolism. The lumbar spine is especially vulnerable, with the majority of herniation occurring at the L4–L5 and L5–S1 levels [11,12]. Pathologically, DDD results from either acute rupture and protrusion of intervertebral disc material or progressive deterioration of surrounding ligamentous and supportive tissues [13]. As demonstrated by the aforementioned clinical cases, the spine's critical role as the body's central skeletal axis—mediating the biomechanical relationship between the upper and lower limbs, has a profound impact on overall health and optimal physical function [14,15]. The peak incidence of intervertebral disc herniation occurs most frequently between the ages of 30 and 50, representing the most vulnerable demographic [16]. Clinically, this condition typically presents as radiating back pain that characteristically extends to the knees, hips, and legs, with symptoms notably exacerbated during Valsalva maneuvers such as sneezing and coughing [17]. Anatomical studies consistently identify the L4–L5 and L5–S1 intervertebral discs as the most common sites of pathological involvement, accounting for the majority of DDD cases [18].

For patients with chronic lumbar DDD, strengthening spinal muscles through supervised physiotherapy and well-designed exercise regimens is essential to mitigate deformity progression [19]. Contemporary rehabilitation paradigms reflect an evolved understanding of exercise-related outcomes. While earlier clinical studies advocated generalized exercise regimens, most notably Williams' flexion exercises, for managing low back pain, more recent biomechanical analyses have demonstrated that such flexion-based protocols may inadvertently increase intervertebral disc pressure, potentially exacerbating the spinal load and compromising structural integrity. This evidence has contributed to a decline in the clinical use of Williams' protocols, with current practice favoring isometric alternatives [20]. Three evidence-based approaches currently dominate clinical practice: (1) static core stabilization targeting deep segmental muscles [21]; (2) integrated strength and endurance training to restore spinal function [22,23]; and (3) individualized protocols tailored to patient-specific pathology.

Rehabilitation programs are essential for both prevention and management of LBP and require individualised planning and close supervision by trained specialists. Optimal outcomes depend on tailoring exercise selection and program design to the specific DDD subtype (e.g., classified by location, such as cervical or lumbar, degeneration patterns like disc space narrowing, or the presence of features such as osteophyte formation) and the individual symptom profile. Evidence suggests that individualized rehabilitation not only alleviates current symptoms but also reduces recurrence, thereby improving quality of life [14,24]. To address gaps in current rehabilitation practices, this systematic review evaluates the efficacy of exercise-based interventions for lumbar DDD, with an emphasis on identifying strategies for pain relief and secondary prevention.

2. Materials and Methods

This systematic review, conducted in 2025, evaluates the therapeutic effects of various exercise interventions within a rehabilitation framework for lumbar DDD.

Following established methodological standards, we utilised the Preferred Reporting Items for Systematic Reviews and Meta-Analyses (PRISMA) guidelines to conduct this comprehensive review [25]. Our systematic process adhered to the standard PRISMA framework, comprising four key phases: (1) initial article identification through database searches, (2) rigorous screening of potential studies, (3) detailed eligibility assessment, and (4) final inclusion of qualifying articles. The full flow of this selection process, including the number of studies identified and excluded at each stage, is illustrated in the PRISMA diagram (Figure 1). The review protocol was registered with the International Prospective Register of Systematic Reviews (PROSPERO) under registration number CRD420251088811.

2.1. Search Strategy

A comprehensive systematic search was conducted across six electronic databases: three international (PubMed, Web of Science, Scopus) and three regional Persian-language databases (Magiran, Noormags, and SID).

Additionally, the Google Scholar search engine was queried to ensure thorough coverage of grey literature. The search covered the period from 1 January 2010 to 1 January 2025. Keywords were selected based on established MeSH terms, a review of relevant literature, and pilot searches to optimize sensitivity. The search terms were organized into two main concepts: (1) the population (i.e., lumbar degenerative disc disease) and (2) the intervention (i.e., exercise-based rehabilitation). The intervention keywords were intentionally expanded to include a broad range of modalities such as Pilates, yoga, aquatic therapy, and suspension training to ensure a comprehensive search.

The Boolean operators "AND" (to combine the two main concepts) and "OR" (to combine keywords within each concept) were used. This logical framework was systematically adapted to meet the specific syntax requirements of each database, ensuring a consistent and comprehensive search. For full transparency and reproducibility, the complete search strings used for PubMed, Scopus, Web of Science, and Google Scholar are provided in Supplementary File S1. Equivalent Persian-language keywords were applied for the regional Persian databases. To further ensure comprehensive literature coverage, the reference lists of all included articles were also manually screened using a snowballing method.

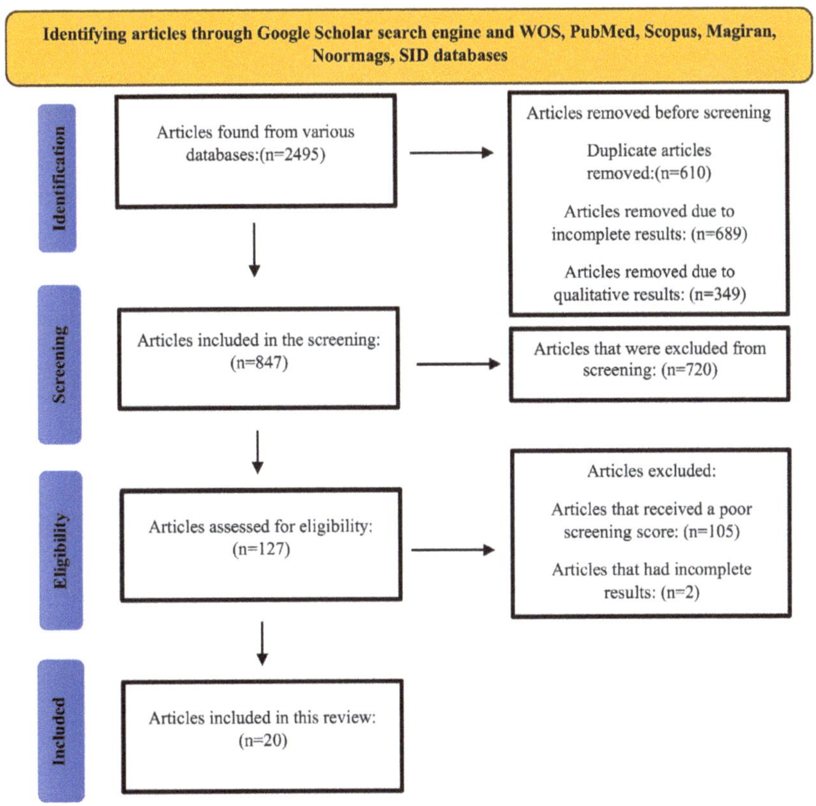

Figure 1. The process of searching, reviewing, and selecting articles based on the PRISMA guidelines.

2.2. Eligibility Criteria and Study Selection

Inclusion criteria were established prior to data extraction to guide the systematic review process. The primary selection criteria focused on studies evaluating the effects of various exercise-based rehabilitation interventions for lumbar DDD. Eligible studies met the following requirements: (1) full-text availability in English or Persian, (2) clinical trial design, and (3) inclusion of human participants to assess the practical efficacy of exercise interventions. Exclusion criteria eliminated studies addressing acute low back pain, specific etiologies of LBP, and those investigating combined treatment protocols (e.g., exercise plus pharmacological therapy) for nonspecific chronic LBP. Studies involving comorbid conditions—such as multiple sclerosis or pregnancy—were also excluded.

The initial screening of titles and abstracts, followed by full-text assessment, was conducted independently by two reviewers (S.A. and F.R.). Any disagreements were resolved by consensus or, if necessary, through consultation with a third reviewer (F.I.). A rigorous screening process was applied after implementing the inclusion and exclusion criteria. The included studies were categorized into two main groups: (1) conventional rehabilitation methods and (2) specialized sports-oriented approaches. These studies were analyzed based on intervention types, exercise outcomes, expert perspectives, muscle electromyographic (EMG) activity, and instrumentation, with findings presented through both textual descriptions and tables.

Participant groups across studies included athletes and non-athletes, with no restrictions on age or gender. Outcomes examined included the effects of suspension training on EMG activity, plantar pressure distribution patterns, and comparisons of diagnostic methods in clinical settings.

2.3. Data Extraction

A standardized data extraction form was developed to systematically collect relevant information from all included studies. Two review authors (F.I. and S.A.), both with extensive experience in rehabilitation and systematic review methodologies, independently extracted the data. The extracted information included: (1) study characteristics (first author, year of publication, study design); (2) participant details (sample size, age, gender); (3) intervention characteristics (type, duration, frequency); and (4) primary outcome measures and key quantitative results. Any disagreements between the two reviewers were initially resolved through discussion to reach consensus. If consensus could not be achieved, a third senior reviewer (F.R.) was consulted to arbitrate and make the final decision.

2.4. Quality Appraisal

The methodological quality of the included studies was independently assessed by two authors (F.I. and M.N.S.) using the McMaster Critical Review Form for Quantitative Studies [26]. This standardized tool comprises 17 distinct criteria designed to systematically evaluate key aspects of research methodology. Specifically, it assesses the clarity of study objectives, appropriateness of the research design, sampling rigor, validity of outcome measures, intervention protocols, statistical analyses, and the validity of conclusions.

The quality assessment followed the standardised McMaster Review Guide, specifically developed for quantitative research (Table 1). Each item was scored dichotomously: a score of "1" indicated full adherence to the criterion, while a score of "0" reflected non-fulfillment.

Total scores were summed to determine methodological quality and categorized as follows: Poor (0–8), Average (9–10), Good (11–12), Very Good (13–14), and Excellent (15–16).

2.5. Data Synthesis and Analysis

Due to significant heterogeneity among the included studies in terms of intervention protocols and outcome measures, a meta-analysis was deemed inappropriate. This heterogeneity was evident across multiple domains: interventions varied widely, ranging from manual therapies (e.g., massage) and mind–body exercises (e.g., yoga, Pilates) to facility-based programs (e.g., aquatic therapy, suspension training).

Furthermore, the studies utilised a wide array of outcome measures, including the Visual Analogue Scale (VAS), the Oswestry Disability Index, and various biomechanical tests, which prevented statistical pooling of the results. Finally, the intervention protocols varied significantly in duration and frequency. Given this high level of clinical and methodological variability, a narrative synthesis was conducted to summarize and describe the findings.

Table 1. Items and descriptions from the McMaster Critical Review Questionnaire for Quantitative Studies.

Item	Description
1	**Objective**: Was the purpose clearly stated?
2	**Literature review**: Was relevant background literature reviewed?
3	**Study design**: What type of study design was used?
4	**Sample size justification**: Was the sample size determination explained?
5	**Sample description**: Was the sample described in detail?
6	**Outcome reliability**: Were the outcome measures reliable?
7	**Outcome validity**: Were the outcome measures valid?
8	**Intervention details**: Was the intervention described in sufficient detail?
9	**Contamination**: Was contamination prevented?
10	**Co-intervention**: Were co-interventions avoided?
11	**Statistical significance**: Were statistically significant results reported?
12	**Statistical analysis**: Were the analytical methods appropriate?
13	**Clinical significance**: Was clinical significance reported?
14	**Withdrawal criteria**: Were withdrawal criteria reported?
15	**Conclusions**: Were conclusions appropriate given the methods and results?
16	**Clinical implications**: Were clinical implications of the findings discussed?
17	**Study limitations**: Were major study limitations or biases reported?

3. Results

3.1. Study Selection

Our systematic search initially identified 2495 potentially relevant articles through keyword searches. After removing duplicates, 1847 articles remained. Following title and abstract screening, 1720 studies were excluded. The full texts of the remaining 127 articles were assessed for eligibility, which resulted in the exclusion of a further 107 studies. The primary reasons for exclusion at this stage were insufficient methodological quality (n = 105) and incomplete results (n = 2). Ultimately, 20 studies met the full inclusion criteria and were included in this systematic review. The complete flow of the study selection process is illustrated in the PRISMA diagram (Figure 1).

3.2. Study Characteristics and Methodological Quality

The 20 included studies encompassed a variety of research designs: seven were clinical trials, seven were semi-experimental or applied designs, three were experimental, two were descriptive, and one was a quasi-experimental study. The participant populations included both males and females with ages ranging from 20 to 83 years. Sample sizes in the studies varied, ranging from 14 to 453 participants. The methodological quality of the included articles, assessed using the McMaster questionnaire, was varied. Eight studies were rated as "excellent" quality, seven as "very good" quality, and five as "good" quality. A detailed breakdown of the quality assessment scores for each study is presented in Table 2.

Table 2. Quality assessment results based on McMaster's critical questionnaire.

Author/Year	1	2	3	4	5	6	7	8	9	10	11	12	13	14	15	16	17	Total Score
Sobhani et al. (2023) [27]	1	1	1	1	1	1	1	1	1	0	1	1	1	1	1	1	1	16/16
Dehmordi & Fattahi (2022) [28]	1	1	1	1	0	1	1	1	1	1	1	0	1	1	1	0	0	13/16
Alhamashi et al. (2022) [29]	1	1	1	1	1	1	1	1	N/A	1	1	1	0	1	1	0	1	14/15
Mohebbi Rad et al. (2022) [30]	1	1	1	1	1	1	1	1	1	1	1	1	0	1	1	0	0	14/15
Mohebbi Rad et al. (2022) (2) [31]	1	1	1	1	1	1	1	1	1	1	1	1	1	1	1	1	0	16/16
Mohebbi Rad et al. (2022) (3) [32]	1	1	1	1	1	1	1	1	1	1	1	1	0	1	1	0	0	14/16
Gandomi et al. (2021) [33]	1	1	1	1	1	1	1	1	1	1	1	1	0	1	1	0	0	14/16
Hawrylak et al. (2021) [34]	1	1	1	0	1	1	1	1	1	1	1	1	1	1	1	1	1	16/16
Ezadi et al. (2021) [35]	1	1	1	0	1	1	0	1	1	1	1	1	1	1	0	0	0	12/16
Kałużna et al. (2019) [36]	1	1	1	0	0	1	1	0	1	1	1	1	1	0	1	0	0	11/16
Mostaghel et al. (2019) [18]	1	1	1	0	1	1	1	1	1	1	1	1	1	0	1	1	0	14/16
Lizis et al. (2017) [37]	1	1	1	0	1	1	1	1	1	1	1	1	1	1	1	1	1	16/16
Ghorbani et al. (2018) [38]	1	1	1	0	0	1	1	1	1	0	1	1	0	1	1	0	0	11/16
Ilbeigi et al. (2018) [39]	1	1	1	0	1	1	1	1	1	1	1	1	1	0	1	1	1	15/16
Teherán et al. (2016) [40]	1	1	1	0	1	1	1	1	1	1	1	1	0	1	1	1	1	15/16
Lotfi et al. (2015) [41]	1	1	1	0	1	1	1	0	1	1	1	1	1	0	1	0	0	12/16
Nazemzadeh et al. (2013) [42]	1	1	1	0	1	1	1	0	1	1	1	1	1	0	1	1	1	14/16
Dzierżanowski et al. (2013) [4]	1	1	1	0	1	1	1	1	N/A	1	1	1	1	0	1	1	1	14/15
Khanzadeh et al. (2012) [43]	1	1	1	0	1	1	1	1	1	1	1	0	1	1	1	1	0	14/16
Akbari & Rezaei (2011) [44]	1	1	1	0	1	1	1	1	1	1	1	1	0	1	0	0	1	13/16
Total Studies Meeting Criterion (n = 20)	20	20	20	7	17	20	19	17	18	18	20	18	13	14	18	10	9	-

1 = Criteria Fully Met, 0 = Criteria Not Fully Met. Quality Categories: Poor (0–8), Average (9–10), Good (11–12), Very Good (13–14), and Excellent (15–16). N/A: "Not applicable" was used for Item 9 (Contamination) only in single-group studies where the criterion was not relevant; for these studies, the denominator for the total score was adjusted to 15.

3.3. Intervention Characteristics

The interventions varied significantly across the studies. Core stability exercises were the most common intervention (20%). Other prominent interventions included combined exercise and massage protocols (15%); suspension exercises, yoga, and Pilates (15%); aquatic exercises (10%); and massage therapy alone (10%). The duration of interventions typically ranged from 2 to 8 weeks, with frequencies of two to four sessions per week. Session durations generally ranged from 20 to 60 min. While a few studies reported intensity using subjective measures like the Borg scale, none of the included studies reported standardized, objective information on the intensity of the interventions. Details of each intervention protocol are summarized in Table 3.

Table 3. (**A**) Study Characteristics. (**B**) Intervention Protocols and Outcomes.

(A)								
Authors	**Study Objectives**	**Research Design**	**Population/Sample Size/Gender/Age**	**Intervention Duration**	**Frequency**	**Session Duration (min)**	**Intervention Intensity**	**Equipment**
Sobhani et al. (2024) [27]	Effectiveness of 8-week motor control retraining on chronic LBP in military males with lumbar disc herniation	Randomized Controlled Trial (RCT)	36 military males (intervention /control groups) /42.88 ± 7.96 years	8 weeks	3 sessions /week	45–60	NR	Electrotherapy
Dehmordi & Fattahi (2023) [28]	Effects of 6-week Pilates on disability and core metrics in women with lumbar disc herniation	Quasi-experimental (pre-post with control group)	30 women (15/15 groups)/ 55.6 ± 4.3 years	6 weeks	3 sessions /week	60	NR	Exercise equipment

Table 3. *Cont.*

(A)								
Authors	**Study Objectives**	**Research Design**	**Population/Sample Size/Gender/Age**	**Intervention Duration**	**Frequency**	**Session Duration (min)**	**Intervention Intensity**	**Equipment**
Alhamashi et al. (2022) [29]	Short-term massage effects on plantar pressure and pain in women with discogenic LBP	Quasi-experimental (single-group pre-post)	14 women/ 35–45 years	5 sessions	Daily	15	NR	Force plate
Mohebbi Rad et al. (2021) [30]	Suspension training effects on EMG in men with chronic LBP from disc herniation	Non-Randomized Clinical Trial	22 men (12 suspension/ 10 control)/ 34.25 ± 8.81 years	8 weeks	3 sessions /week	30	Borg scale up to 6	EMG device
Mohebbi Rad et al. (2021) [31]	Comparison of core stability vs. suspension training on β-endorphins and pain	Non-Randomized Clinical Trial	32 men (10 core/ 12 suspension/ 10 control)/ 25–45 years	8 weeks	3 sessions /week	30	Borg scale: 5 (Core), 6 (Suspension)	BEURER scale, ZELL BIO kit
Mohebbi Rad et al. (2021) [32]	Effects 8-week core stability on abdominal muscle activation	Non-Randomized Clinical Trial	20 men (10/10 groups)/ 20–50 years	8 weeks	3 sessions /week	30	Borg scale up to 5	EMG device
Gandomi et al. (2021) [33]	Plantar pressure distribution patterns in women with discogenic LBP	Descriptive	34 women (17 LBP/ 17 healthy)/ Mean 63 years	N/A	N/A	N/A	N/A	PT scan device
Hawrylak et al. (2021) [34]	McKenzie method efficacy for lumbar DDD	Experimental (pre-post with control group)	60 patients (40–59 years)	2 weeks (10 session)	Daily (weekdays)	30	NR	Digital inclinometer
Ezadi & Ghanizadeh Hesar (2021) [35]	Aquatic exercises' effects on pain/balance in nurses with chronic LBP	Quasi-experimental (pre-post with control group)	30 female nurses (15/15 groups)/ 25–40 years	8 weeks	3 sessions /week	NR	NR	-
Kałużna et al. (2019) [36]	Stabilization exercises for lumbar DDD	Experimental (pre-post with control group)	30 patients (16F/14M)/ 25–68 years	14 days	NR	NR	NR	-
Mostaghel et al. (2019) [18]	Acupuncture + aquatic exercise for DDD	Quasi-experimental (comparative design)	24 women (12/12 groups)	8 weeks	3 sessions /week	45–60	NR	-
Latafatkar et al. (2018) [38]	Stability exercises vs. reflexology for chronic LBP	Quasi-experimental (multi-group design)	47 women (4 groups)/ 30–35 years	8 weeks	3 sessions /week	15–30	NR	-
Ilbeigi et al. (2018) [39]	Kinesiotaping vs. foot reflexology for non-specific LBP	Quasi-experimental (multi-group design)	30 men (3 groups)/ 20–40 years	6 weeks	3 sessions /week	30	NR	-
Lizis et al. (2017) [37]	Kaltenborn-Evjenth Orthopaedic Manual Therapy (KEOMT) vs. kinesiotherapy for DDD	Randomized Controlled Trial (RCT)	80 patients (40–70 years)	5 weeks (10 treatments)	2 sessions /week	30 (KEOMT), 45 (Kinesiotherapy)	NR	Kinesiotape

Table 3. *Cont.*

(A)								
Authors	**Study Objectives**	**Research Design**	**Population/Sample Size/Gender/Age**	**Intervention Duration**	**Frequency**	**Session Duration (min)**	**Intervention Intensity**	**Equipment**
Teherán et al. (2016) [40]	Alternative therapies for lumbar disc disease	Descriptive, Retrospective Study	453 patients/ Mean 57 years	Variable (>6 months)	N/A	N/A	N/A	-
Lotfi et al. (2016) [41]	Supine aquatic exercises for men with discogenic LBP	Quasi-experimental (pre-post with control group)	24 men (12/12 groups)/ Mean 38.83 ± 5.78 years	6 weeks (24 sessions)	4 sessions /week	45–60	NR	-
Nazemzadeh et al. (2013) [42]	Foot reflexology physiological effects	Randomized Controlled Trial (RCT)	150 men (3 groups)/ 45.8 ± 13.39 years	3 weeks	1 session /week	30	NR	Sphygmomanometer
Dzierżanowski et al. (2013) [4]	Low-position exercises for lumbar-sacral DDD	Experimental (single-group pre-post)	20 patients (17F/3M)/ 24–73 years	2 weeks (10 days)	Daily (week-days)	20	NR	-
Khanzadeh et al. (2012) [43]	Combined exercise + massage protocol	Quasi-experimental (pre-post with control group)	30 men (15/15 groups) /41.61 ± 4.98 years	8 weeks	3 sessions /week	60	NR	-
Akbari & Rezaei (2012) [44]	Yoga effects on flexibility/pain in chronic disc herniation	Double-Blind Randomized Controlled Trial (RCT)	28 women (14/14 groups)/ 30–40 years	8 weeks (16 sessions)	2 sessions /week	45	NR	Flexible ruler

(B)			
Authors	**Researchprotocol**	**Results**	**Conclusions**
Sobhani et al. (2024) [27]	Functional disability questionnaire, VAS pain scale	• Significant improvements in pain intensity ($p < 0.05$), functional disability, and range of motion.	• Motor control retraining effectively improves pain, disability, and ROM, and may enhance QoL in military personnel.
Dehmordi & Fattahi (2023) [28]	Oswestry Disability Index, Schober test, Pilates tests	• 6 weeks of Pilates significantly improved disability, trunk flexibility, and core muscle strength/endurance.	• Pilates rehabilitation is a recommended intervention for symptom management in patients with lumbar disc herniation.
Alhamashi et al. (2022) [29]	Plantar pressure assessment and pain intensity evaluation	• Significant pain reduction was observed after 5 massage sessions. • Plantar pressure improved significantly after 5 sessions, but not after a single session.	• While a single massage session can reduce pain, five sessions may be needed to influence compensatory mechanisms related to plantar pressure.
Mohebbi Rad et al. (2021) [30]	EMG assessment and straight leg lowering test	• Suspension group showed significant improvement in EMG activity of four muscles and strength test performance compared to controls.	• Suspension training enhances core muscle activation and is a valuable component of rehabilitation programs.
Mohebbi Rad et al. (2021) [31]	Core stability and suspension training protocols	• Both exercise types improved β-endorphin, pain, and disability. • Suspension training demonstrated superior pain and disability reduction compared to core stability.	• Suspension training appears more effective for pain and disability management in lumbar disc herniation patients.
Mohebbi Rad et al. (2021) [32]	EMG activity, abdominal strength, and flexibility tests	• 8 weeks of core stability training led to significant improvements in muscle activation, strength, and flexibility.	• Core stability exercises lead to notable improvements in trunk muscle function and should be included in rehabilitation.

Table 3. *Cont.*

(B)			
Authors	**Researchprotocol**	**Results**	**Conclusions**
Gandomi et al. (2021) [33]	Center of pressure and symmetry index assessment	• Disc herniation patients showed significant increases in sway velocity and path length, and reduced symmetry, compared to controls.	• Neuromuscular training for spinal stabilizers may help reduce subsequent injury risk in this population.
Hawrylak et al. (2021) [34]	Conservative McKenzie physiotherapy method	• Both the McKenzie and standard physiotherapy groups improved, but enhanced outcomes were observed in the McKenzie group.	• The McKenzie method is a clinically useful intervention for lumbar DDD management.
Ezadi & Gha-nizadeh Hesar (2021) [35]	Stork test, Berg test, Quebec Disability Scale	• The aquatic exercise group showed significant pain reduction and balance improvement compared to the control group.	• Aquatic exercise protocols focusing on core muscle strengthening should be emphasized in therapeutic programs.
Kałużna et al. (2019) [36]	Functional Movement Screen (FMS), VAS pain scale	• Deep muscle stabilization exercises significantly reduced lumbar pain and positively affected global movement patterns.	• Stabilization exercises positively impact pain reduction and functional status in patients with lumbar DDD.
Mostaghel et al. (2019) [18]	VAS, Straight Leg Raise test, SF-36 questionnaire	• 8 weeks of combined acupuncture and aquatic exercise led to significant improvements in pain, ROM, and quality of life.	• Both acupuncture and aquatic exercise are effective for pain reduction, mobility improvement, and quality of life.
Latafatkar et al. (2018) [38]	McGill functional tests, VAS pain scale	• Stability exercises (alone and combined) improved muscle endurance and pain with durable effects. • Reflexology massage only showed positive effects on pain reduction.	• Due to their durable effects, core stability exercises should be prioritized in chronic LBP treatment protocols.
Ilbeigi et al. (2018) [39]	VAS pain scale, Oswestry Disability Index	• Both kinesiotaping and foot reflexology reduced pain and disability. • Kinesiotaping showed significantly greater pain reduction than reflexology.	• While both methods are effective, kinesiotaping may be preferable for achieving greater pain relief.
Lizis et al. (2017) [37]	SF-36 quality of life form, VAS pain scale	• After 5 weeks, KEOMT showed statistically significant advantages over kinesiotherapy for all QoL domains and pain.	• KEOMT is more effective than kinesiotherapy for improving quality of life and pain in lumbar DDD patients.
Teherán et al. (2016) [40]	Alternative therapy evaluation	• Alternative therapies demonstrated a 50–60-point pain reduction, sustained for over 6 months.	• Alternative therapies show significant impact on chronic pain in patients unresponsive to conventional treatments.
Lotfi et al. (2016) [41]	Aquatic movement therapy, Student's t-test	• The aquatic exercise group showed significant reductions in pain intensity and greater disability reduction compared to the control group.	• Supine aquatic exercises can effectively reduce pain and functional disability in men with chronic discogenic LBP.
Nazemzadeh et al. (2013) [42]	Physiological measures (respiratory rate, pulse, BP)	• Post-intervention, all three groups (intervention, placebo, control) showed reduced respiratory rate and blood pressure.	• Foot reflexology may effectively improve physiological indicators in LBP patients, suggesting clinical utility.

Table 3. *Cont.*

(B)			
Authors	**Researchprotocol**	**Results**	**Conclusions**
Dzierżanowski et al. (2013) [4]	Schober test, finger-to-floor test, seated spinal rotation	• 90% of patients reported improved lateral spinal flexion after 2 weeks of rehabilitation.	• Active low-position exercises significantly improve range of motion, postural alignment, and pain reduction.
Khanzadeh et al. (2012) [43]	Combined exercise and massage protocol	• The experimental group showed significant improvements in physical function and pain scores after 8 weeks.	• A combined exercise and massage protocol is an effective approach for improving function and reducing pain.
Akbari & Rezaei (2012) [44]	VAS, Oswestry Disability Index, Beck Depression Inventory	• Both yoga and conventional exercises significantly reduced pain, disability, depression, and lordosis, and improved ROM. • No significant differences were found between the two interventions.	• Yoga and conventional exercises show comparable effectiveness for managing symptoms in women with chronic lumbar disc herniation.

Notes: N/A: Not applicable, NR: Not reported.

3.4. Main Outcomes

All 20 included studies reported positive outcomes, demonstrating that exercise-based rehabilitation is an effective strategy for managing lumbar DDD. Key findings from specific modalities include:

Aquatic exercises showed multiple benefits, including pain reduction, improved static and dynamic balance, increased range of motion, enhanced quality of life, and decreased disability.

Core stability exercises, comprising 20% of the studied interventions, showed comprehensive benefits. These benefits included reductions in pain intensity and functional disability, increases in range of motion and trunk flexibility, as well as improvements in core muscle endurance and performance.

In a direct comparison, one study found that suspension training was more effective than isolated core stability exercises in reducing pain (mean difference: −1.74; $p < 0.001$) and disability (mean difference: −8.21; $p < 0.001$).

Massage therapy, reported in 10% of the studies, significantly reduced pain but did not improve muscle endurance. Additionally, reflexology interventions were effective in alleviating pain, and some manual therapies demonstrated improvements in plantar pressure distribution. Other interventions, such as yoga and conventional rehabilitation programs, were also found to be effective. For example, yoga showed comparable effectiveness to conventional exercises in reducing pain and disability.

The McKenzie method also proved effective, with one trial demonstrating statistically significant advantages ($p < 0.001$) in improving spinal mobility and reducing pain compared to standard physiotherapy.

Comparative studies evaluated different modalities. For instance, one study comparing acupuncture and aquatic exercise found both interventions to be effective in improving pain, mobility, and quality of life, with no significant differences between them.

4. Discussion

The primary aim of this study was to systematically analyze the therapeutic effects of various rehabilitation exercises on lumbar DDD and to identify the most effective methods for preventing and alleviating back pain in affected individuals. The synthesis of the

20 included studies confirms the overall efficacy of exercise-based rehabilitation but also suggests a potential hierarchy of effectiveness among different modalities. Notably, the evidence indicates that dynamic and multi-component interventions may produce superior outcomes; for instance, a clinical trial by Mohebbi Rad et al. (2021) demonstrated that suspension training was more effective than isolated core stability exercises in reducing both pain (mean difference: −1.74) and disability (mean difference: −8.21), Aquatic therapy consistently demonstrated broad benefits across pain reduction, functional improvement, and balance [31]. This suggests that while most exercise-based approaches are beneficial, the choice of intervention can be tailored to target specific clinical goals.

The clinical benefits of hydrotherapy are multifaceted, primarily resulting from three key physiological mechanisms: substantial reduction of weight-bearing forces, enhanced sensation of lightness and fluid movement in the aquatic environment, and significant decrease in mechanical loading on articular structures. Additionally, the combined effects of hydrostatic weightlessness and the inherent massage-like properties of water immersion have been scientifically shown to produce measurable therapeutic outcomes, including notable reduction or complete resolution of muscle cramps and subsequent alleviation of disc-related muscular spasms [45,46].

Lotfi et al. [41] conducted a study investigating the effects of aquatic therapy, specifically examining how six weeks of supine water exercises impacted pain severity and disability levels in male patients with chronic low back pain due to lumbar disc herniation. Their results demonstrated statistically significant reductions in both pain intensity and disability within the experimental group, clearly indicating that aquatic exercise programs can effectively improve clinical outcomes in patients with lumbar pathologies.

Building on these findings, Mostaghel et al. [18] conducted a comparative study evaluating the effects of eight weeks of combined acupuncture and aquatic exercise therapy in patients with lumbar DDD. Their research assessed multiple outcomes, including pain levels, range of motion, and quality of life improvements. While both treatment modalities demonstrated comparable effectiveness in reducing pain, enhancing mobility, and improving quality of life, the study found no significant differences between the acupuncture and aquatic exercise groups, suggesting that either approach could be effectively incorporated into treatment protocols.

Further supporting evidence comes from Ezadi et al. [35], who implemented an eight-week program of selected aquatic exercises in a quasi-experimental study involving thirty female nurses with chronic low back pain from Sanandaj hospitals. Their results revealed significant between-group differences, with the intervention group demonstrating marked reductions in pain scores and clinically meaningful improvements in both static and dynamic balance measures. These positive outcomes were not observed in the control group, reinforcing aquatic exercise as an evidence-based intervention for enhancing motor function and alleviating pain in patients with lumbar DDD. Collectively, these studies position aquatic therapy as a particularly robust intervention due to its consistent, multi-domain benefits—including pain relief, balance enhancement, and improved quality of life—a breadth of effect not always achieved by more targeted, land-based exercises.

The collective results consistently identify stability exercises as an effective rehabilitation method, with documented improvements in both patient function and pain reduction. Clinical observations indicate altered movement patterns and impaired activation of the deep back muscles—the primary stabilizers of the lumbar region—in patients with chronic nonspecific low back pain [47,48].

These neuromuscular changes frequently contribute to pain development, muscular imbalances, and subsequent functional impairments, thereby reinforcing the therapeutic rationale for implementing stability exercises in both pain management and performance recovery [49].

Further supporting evidence is provided by Gandomi et al. [33], who specifically investigated plantar pressure distribution patterns, symmetry indices, and center of pressure fluctuations in female patients with discogenic low back pain. Their comparative analysis revealed significant differences in both pressure metrics and postural fluctuations between the disc herniation group and healthy controls, underscoring the critical role of core stability exercises in enhancing balance and motor control within this population.

Mohebbi Rad et al. [31] contributed to this body of evidence by directly comparing core stability exercises with suspension exercises in patients with lumbar disc herniation. Their findings showed that although both intervention groups achieved significant clinical improvements, the suspension exercise group experienced superior outcomes in terms of pain reduction and functional disability. These results were further supported by a follow-up study conducted by Mohebbi Rad et al. [32], which assessed electromyographic activity and reported markedly enhanced muscle activation patterns in the suspension exercise group, thereby providing physiological evidence for the effectiveness of suspension exercise interventions in improving physical function. This highlights a key theme in modern rehabilitation: while isolated core stability exercises form a foundational component, progression to more dynamic and challenging protocols, such as suspension training, may be necessary to maximize gains in pain relief and functional improvement.

Dzierżanowski et al. [4] investigated the effects of active exercises performed in low positions on lumbosacral function in patients with DDD. Their findings demonstrated that this specific exercise approach offers multiple clinical benefits: it significantly enhances the range of motion in the affected region, improves postural alignment, and reduces lower back pain. Moreover, these exercises led to measurable improvements in patients' functional capacity for daily activities, highlighting their practical relevance in rehabilitation settings.

The accumulated body of evidence strongly supports the therapeutic value of aquatic exercise and complementary interventions for musculoskeletal disorders [42,43]. In light of these findings, we recommend integrating these modalities into comprehensive physiotherapy and multidisciplinary treatment programs for patients with spinal conditions. Emphasis should be placed on further research and the clinical implementation of these approaches. Several key findings support this recommendation: deep muscle training programs have demonstrated significant efficacy in alleviating back pain [50]; targeted exercise interventions effectively improve dysfunctional movement patterns [51]; and although some studies reported no significant differences between experimental and control groups in perceived pain or FMS scores, our review indicates that regular physical activity consistently leads to improved functional outcomes. Collectively, these findings reinforce the importance of exercise-based rehabilitation while emphasising the need for personalised treatment plans that account for individual patient characteristics.

The review also found that other modalities, while effective, generally demonstrated comparable rather than superior outcomes. For example, yoga was found to be as effective as conventional exercise, and manual therapies such as massage significantly reduced pain but did not improve muscle endurance. These findings suggest that for specific patient profiles or treatment goals, multiple viable options exist, with intervention selection potentially guided by patient preference and clinical presentation.

Despite the valuable insights provided by this systematic review, several limitations must be acknowledged. First, considerable heterogeneity was observed among the included studies in terms of intervention protocols—particularly regarding duration, intensity, and frequency—which complicates direct comparisons and precludes meta-analytic synthesis. Second, many trials enrolled fewer than 30 participants, a sample size widely recognized as underpowered for detecting moderate clinical effects, potentially limiting statistical power and the generalizability of findings [11,52]. Third, the current evidence base lacks robust longitudinal data, as most studies did not include long-term follow-up, thereby restricting the assessment of the durability of therapeutic effects. Consequently, while clinicians can confidently recommend these exercise interventions for short-term pain relief, their efficacy in preventing long-term recurrence remains uncertain.

Furthermore, our methodological quality appraisal revealed that the majority of studies were of high quality: 75% (15 out of 20) of the studies received an "excellent" or "very good" rating on the McMaster scale. However, the remaining variability suggests the potential for bias in outcome reporting. A closer examination of the quality appraisal (Table 2) revealed that the most prevalent methodological limitations among the included studies were the absence of sample size justification and inadequate reporting of participant withdrawal criteria.

Consequently, while the findings from studies with lower quality scores (e.g., Ghorbani et al. [38]; Kałużna et al. [36]) are included in our narrative synthesis, their contribution to the overall evidence should be interpreted with greater caution. Several studies also utilized quasi-experimental designs without random assignment, which increases susceptibility to selection bias, maturation effects, and other threats to internal validity [53,54]. Furthermore, the potential for publication bias—where studies reporting positive results are more likely to be published than those with null findings—cannot be excluded and may result in an overestimation of the true effect of these interventions. Lastly, although our search strategy was comprehensive, limiting the review to articles published in English and Persian may have led to the omission of relevant studies published in other languages.

Taken together, these limitations highlight an urgent need for future research involving larger, adequately powered randomised controlled trials (e.g., based on a priori power analyses to detect clinically meaningful effects, e.g., with sample sizes exceeding 100 participants per arm), standardised intervention protocols, and extended follow-up durations of at least 12 months post-intervention to better establish the long-term efficacy and generalizability of exercise-based rehabilitation for lumbar DDD.

5. Conclusions

This systematic review demonstrates that rehabilitation exercises, including hydrotherapy, core stability training, Pilates, and suspension exercises, effectively reduce pain and improve function in patients with lumbar DDD. The synthesized evidence suggests that when used as primary interventions, multi-component approaches like aquatic therapy and dynamic challenges like suspension training show particularly strong and broad benefits. Based on these findings, we recommend that clinicians consider prioritizing these modalities, especially for patients with significant functional deficits. While one study found no significant difference when combining aquatic therapy with another modality (acupuncture), this does not diminish its overall effectiveness as a core therapeutic strategy. However, it is crucial to acknowledge the limitations of the current evidence base. Therefore, to establish more definitive clinical guidelines, future research should prioritize larger, high-quality randomized controlled trials that employ standardized intervention protocols and include long-term outcome monitoring.

Supplementary Materials: The following supporting information can be downloaded at: https://www.mdpi.com/article/10.3390/healthcare13151938/s1, File S1: PRISMA 2020 Checklist.

Author Contributions: Conceptualization, F.R. and S.A.; methodology, F.R. and F.I.; software, F.I., and M.N.S.; validation, F.R., F.I. and S.A.; formal analysis, F.I. and M.N.S.; investigation, M.N.S. and F.I.; resources, F.R. and G.B.; data curation, F.R. and S.A.; writing—original draft preparation, M.N.S.

and G.B.; writing—review and editing, S.A., F.R., L.P. and F.F.; visualization, G.G.; supervision, L.P., F.F., S.C. and G.G.; project administration, S.C. and G.G. All authors have read and agreed to the published version of the manuscript.

Funding: This research received no external funding.

Institutional Review Board Statement: Not applicable.

Informed Consent Statement: Not applicable.

Conflicts of Interest: The authors declare no conflicts of interest.

Abbreviations

The following abbreviations are used in this manuscript:

DDD	Degenerative disc disease
LBP	Low back pain
YLDs	years lived with disability
PRISMA	Preferred Reporting Items for Systematic Reviews and Meta-Analysis

References

1. Staal, J.B.; Hlobil, H.; Twisk, J.W.; Smid, T.; Köke, A.J.; van Mechelen, W. Graded activity for low back pain in occupational health care: A randomized, controlled trial. *Ann. Intern. Med.* **2004**, *140*, 77–84. [CrossRef]
2. Allegri, M.; Montella, S.; Salici, F.; Valente, A.; Marchesini, M.; Compagnone, C.; Baciarello, M.; Manferdini, M.E.; Fanelli, G. Mechanisms of low back pain: A guide for diagnosis and therapy. *F1000Research* **2016**, *5*, 1530. [CrossRef]
3. Hartvigsen, J.; Hancock, M.J.; Kongsted, A.; Louw, Q.; Ferreira, M.L.; Genevay, S.; Hoy, D.; Karppinen, J.; Pransky, G.; Sieper, J. What low back pain is and why we need to pay attention. *Lancet* **2018**, *391*, 2356–2367. [CrossRef]
4. Dzierżanowski, M.; Dzierżanowski, M.; Maćkowiak, P.; Słomko, W.; Radzimińska, A.; Kaźmierczak, U.; Strojek, K.; Srokowski, G.; Żukow, W. The influence of active exercise in low positions on the functional condition of the lumbar-sacral segment in patients with discopathy. *Adv. Clin. Exp. Med.* **2013**, *22*, 421–430.
5. Harper, W.L.; Schmidt, W.K.; Kubat, N.J.; Isenberg, R.A. An open-label pilot study of pulsed electromagnetic field therapy in the treatment of failed back surgery syndrome pain. *Int. Med. Case Rep. J.* **2014**, *8*, 13–22. [CrossRef]
6. Akuthota, V.; Ferreiro, A.; Moore, T.; Fredericson, M. Core stability exercise principles. *Curr. Sports Med. Rep.* **2008**, *7*, 39–44. [CrossRef] [PubMed]
7. Jegede, K.A.; Ndu, A.; Grauer, J.N. Contemporary management of symptomatic lumbar disc herniations. *Orthop. Clin. Nor. Am.* **2010**, *41*, 217–224. [CrossRef] [PubMed]
8. Cho, K.H.; Beom, J.W.; Lee, T.S.; Lim, J.H.; Lee, T.H.; Yuk, J.H. Trunk muscles strength as a risk factor for nonspecific low back pain: A pilot study. *Ann. Rehabil. Med.* **2014**, *38*, 234–240. [CrossRef]
9. Sharafkhani, N.; Khorsandi, M.; Shamsi, M.; Ranjbaran, M. Low back pain preventive behaviors among nurses based on the health belief model constructs. *SAGE Open* **2014**, *4*, 2158244014556726. [CrossRef]
10. Zanola, R.L.; Donin, C.B.; Bertolini, G.R.F.; Buzanello Azevedo, M.R. Biomechanical repercussion of sitting posture on lumbar intervertebral discs: A systematic review. *J. Bodyw. Mov. Ther.* **2024**, *38*, 384–390. [CrossRef] [PubMed]
11. Billy, G.G.; Lemieux, S.K.; Chow, M.X. Changes in lumbar disk morphology associated with prolonged sitting assessed by magnetic resonance imaging. *PM&R* **2014**, *6*, 790–795. [CrossRef]
12. Al Qaraghli, M.I.; De Jesus, O. Lumbar Disc Herniation. In *StatPearls*; StatPearls: Treasure Island, FL, USA, 2025.
13. Atlas, S.J.; Keller, R.B.; Robson, D.; Deyo, R.A.; Singer, D.E. Surgical and nonsurgical management of lumbar spinal stenosis: Four-year outcomes from the maine lumbar spine study. *Spine* **2000**, *25*, 556–562. [CrossRef]
14. Ferreira, M.L.; Machado, G.; Latimer, J.; Maher, C.; Ferreira, P.H.; Smeets, R.J. Factors defining care-seeking in low back pain–a meta-analysis of population based surveys. *Eur. J. Pain* **2010**, *14*, 747.e1-7. [CrossRef]
15. Demoulin, C.; Crielaard, J.-M.; Vanderthommen, M. Spinal muscle evaluation in healthy individuals and low-back-pain patients: A literature review. *Jt. Bone Spine* **2007**, *74*, 9–13. [CrossRef] [PubMed]
16. Chen, J.; Yang, J.; Ma, L.; Li, J.; Shahzad, N.; Kim, C.K. Structure-antioxidant activity relationship of methoxy, phenolic hydroxyl, and carboxylic acid groups of phenolic acids. *Sci. Rep.* **2020**, *10*, 2611; Erratum in *Sci. Rep.* **2020**, *10*, 5666. [CrossRef] [PubMed]
17. Huang, Y.P.; Bruijn, S.M.; Lin, J.H.; Meijer, O.G.; Wu, W.H.; Abbasi-Bafghi, H.; Lin, X.C.; van Dieën, J.H. Gait adaptations in low back pain patients with lumbar disc herniation: Trunk coordination and arm swing. *Eur. Spine J.* **2011**, *20*, 491–499. [CrossRef]

18. Mostaghel, A.; Salaki, M.; Rahimi, N. Effectiveness of Eight-week Acupuncture and Aquatic Exercise on the Amount of Pain, Motor Range and Quality of Life in Patients with lumbar Discopathy. *Sadra Med. J.* **2019**, *7*, 145–160. [CrossRef]
19. Lee, J.H.; Fell, D.W.; Kim, K. Plantar pressure distribution during walking: Comparison of subjects with and without chronic low back pain. *J. Phys. Ther. Sci.* **2011**, *23*, 923–926. [CrossRef]
20. Hodges, P.W. Core stability exercise in chronic low back pain. *Orthop. Clin. N. Am.* **2003**, *34*, 245–254. [CrossRef] [PubMed]
21. Ramos, L.A.V.; Callegari, B.; França, F.J.R.; Magalhães, M.O.; Burke, T.N.; Carvalho, A.P.d.M.C.; Almeida, G.P.L.; Comachio, J.; Marques, A.P. Comparison between transcutaneous electrical nerve stimulation and stabilization exercises in fatigue and transversus abdominis activation in patients with lumbar disk herniation: A randomized study. *J. Manip. Physiol. Ther.* **2018**, *41*, 323–331. [CrossRef]
22. Bhadauria, E.A.; Gurudut, P. Comparative effectiveness of lumbar stabilization, dynamic strengthening, and Pilates on chronic low back pain: Randomized clinical trial. *J. Exerc. Rehabil.* **2017**, *13*, 477. [CrossRef] [PubMed]
23. Güevenol, K.; Tüzün, Ç.; Peker, Ö.; Göktay, Y. A comparison of inverted spinal traction and conventional traction in the treatment of lumbar disc herniations. *Physiother. Theory Pract.* **2000**, *16*, 151–160. [CrossRef]
24. Wells, C.; Kolt, G.S.; Marshall, P.; Hill, B.; Bialocerkowski, A. The effectiveness of Pilates exercise in people with chronic low back pain: A systematic review. *PLoS ONE* **2014**, *9*, e100402. [CrossRef]
25. Page, M.J.; McKenzie, J.E.; Bossuyt, P.M.; Boutron, I.; Hoffmann, T.C.; Mulrow, C.D.; Shamseer, L.; Tetzlaff, J.M.; Akl, E.A.; Brennan, S.E. The PRISMA 2020 statement: An updated guideline for reporting systematic reviews. *BMJ* **2021**, *372*, 71. [CrossRef] [PubMed]
26. Bhat, I.B.; Najib, A.S.B.M. Hydrotherapy as a Treatment for Non-Specific Low Back Pain: A Systematic Review. *Int. J. Allied Health Sci.* **2023**, *7*, 606–631. [CrossRef]
27. Sobhani, V.; Shirvani, H.; Mehrabian, H.; ebrahim Hashemi, S. Effectiveness of selected Motor Control Retraining Exercises on Chronic Low Back Pain in Male Military Personnel with Lumbar Disc Herniation. A Randomized Controlled Trial. *Asian J. Sports Med.* **2024**, *15*, 1–12. [CrossRef]
28. Mosavi Dehmourdi, L.; Fatahi, H. Effect of Six Weeks of Pilate's Rehabilitation Exercises on Disability, Trunk Flexibility, Core Muscle Strength, and Endurance in Women with Lumber Disc Herniation. *J. Paramed. Sci. Rehabil.* **2023**, *11*, 51–63.
29. Alhamashi, F.; Khoshraftar Yazdi, N.; HashemiJavaheri, A.; Bagheri Mahmudi, M. The Effect of Short Term Massage on Plantar Pressure During Walking and Pain Intensity in Women with Low Back Pain Disc Herniation. *J. Paramed. Sci. Rehabil.* **2022**, *10*, 20–29. [CrossRef]
30. Mohebbi Rad, Y.; Fadaei Chafy, M.R.; Elmieh, A. Effect of Suspension Exercise on Electromyography in Men with Chronic Low Back Pain Caused by Disc Herniation. *J. Maz. Univ. Med. Sci.* **2021**, *31*, 95–104.
31. Mohebbi Rad, Y.; Fadaei Chafy, M.; Elmieh, A. Comparison of the Effect of Core Stability and Suspension Training on Beta Endorphin, Pain, and Functional Disability in Patients with Lumbar Disc Herniation: A Clinical Trial. *J. Rafsanjan Univ. Med. Sci.* **2021**, *20*, 661–680. [CrossRef]
32. Mohebbi Rad, Y.; Fadaei Chafy, M.R.; Elmieh, A. Effect of core stability exercise on activation of abdominal muscles and lumbar flexibility in men with specific chronic low back pain. *Med. J. Mashhad Univ. Med. Sci.* **2021**, *64*, 3047–3059. [CrossRef]
33. Gandomi, F.; Soufivand, P.; Fadaei Dehcheshmeh, P. Studying the pattern of foot pressure distribution, symmetry index, and center of pressure sways in women with back pain due to lumbar disc herniation: A descriptive study. *J. Rafsanjan Univ. Med. Sci.* **2021**, *20*, 487–502. [CrossRef]
34. Hawrylak, A.; Demidaś, A.; Chromik, K.; Hawrylak, A. The effectiveness of the McKenzie method in treating lumbar discopathy. *Human Mov.* **2021**, *22*, 98–104. [CrossRef]
35. Ezadi, H.; Ghanizadeh Hesar, N. The effect of eight weeks of selected exercises in water on pain and balance of female nurses with chronic back pain. *J. Sport Biomech.* **2021**, *7*, 44–55. [CrossRef]
36. Kałużna, A.; Leszczyński, K.; Gałęcki, S.; Płoszaj, O.; Kałużny, K.; Dylewski, M.; Hagner-Derengowska, M.; Zukow, W. The efficiency of stabilization exercises in patients with discopathy in the lumbar spine. *J. Educ. Health Sport* **2019**, *9*, 1043–1050.
37. Lizis, P.; Wiater, S.; Kobza, W. Manual therapy vs. kinesiotherapy for people with lumbar discopathy: A pilot randomized trial. *Rehabil. Sci.* **2017**, *2*, 6–11. [CrossRef]
38. Ghorbani, S.; Letafatkar, A.; Kasbparast, M. Comparison of the effects and durabilities of isolated and combined core stabilization exercise and reflexology massage on muscle endurance and pain in females with chronic non-specific low back pain. *Sci. J. Rehabil. Med.* **2018**, *7*, 90–102. [CrossRef]
39. Ilbeigi, S.; Yaghobi, H.; Mahjur, M.; Seghatoleslamy, A. The comparison of 6 weeks of Kinesio taping and sole reflexology on pain intensity and functional disabilities in male with chronic low back pain. *J. Pract. Stud. Biosci. Sport* **2018**, *5*, 57–66. [CrossRef]
40. Teherán, A.A.; Piñeros, L.G.; Pinilla, L.M.; Borrego, P.; Tijo, A.F.; Mejía, M.C.; Pombo, L.M. Effectiveness of alternative therapies for the management of lumbar disc disease: A descriptive research. *Revista Cuarzo.* **2016**, *22*, 1–12. [CrossRef]
41. Lotfi, H.; Ebrahimi Atri, A.; Hashemi Javaheri, A.; Norouzi, K. The effect of six weeks supine movement in water on the pain and disability in men with chronic low back pain due to lumbar disc herniation. *J. Paramed. Sci. Rehabil.* **2016**, *5*, 14–19. [CrossRef]

42. Zadeh, M.N.; Rezvani, M.; Jalalodini, A.; Navidian, A.; Yosefian, N.; Ghalje, M.; Pournamdar, Z. The effect of reflexology massage on physiological parameters in patients with chronic low back pain. *Pajoohande* **2013**, *17*, 286–290.
43. Khanzadeh, R.; Hashemi, A.A.; Omidi Kashani, F.; Zandi, M.; Khodabakhshi, M. The Effect of Combined Therapeutic Protocol (Therapeutic Exercises and Massage) on the Pain and Physical Performance in Men with Chronic Low Back Pain due to Lumbar Disc Herniation. *Evid. Based Care* **2012**, *2*, 29–36. [CrossRef]
44. Akbari, A.; Rezaei, S. The effect of yoga exercises on lumbar range of motion, pain and functional disability in women with chroniclumbar disk herniation: A randomized controlled study. *J. Ilam. Uni. Med. Sci.* **2012**, *20*, 16–28.
45. Becker, B.E. Aquatic therapy: Scientific foundations and clinical rehabilitation applications. *PM&R* **2009**, *1*, 859–872. [CrossRef]
46. Prins, J.; Cutner, D. Aquatic therapy in the rehabilitation of athletic injuries. *Clin. Sports Med.* **1999**, *18*, 447–461. [CrossRef]
47. Macedo, L.G.; Maher, C.G.; Latimer, J.; McAuley, J.H. Motor control exercise for persistent, nonspecific low back pain: A systematic review. *Phys. Ther.* **2009**, *89*, 9–25. [CrossRef] [PubMed]
48. França, F.R.; Burke, T.N.; Caffaro, R.R.; Ramos, L.A.; Marques, A.P. Effects of muscular stretching and segmental stabilization on functional disability and pain in patients with chronic low back pain: A randomized, controlled trial. *J. Manip. Physiol. Ther.* **2012**, *35*, 279–285. [CrossRef]
49. Mannion, A.; Caporaso, F.; Pulkovski, N.; Sprott, H. Spine stabilisation exercises in the treatment of chronic low back pain: A good clinical outcome is not associated with improved abdominal muscle function. *Eur. Spine J.* **2012**, *21*, 1301–1310. [CrossRef] [PubMed]
50. Paungmali, A.; Joseph, L.H.; Punturee, K.; Sitilertpisan, P.; Pirunsan, U.; Uthaikhup, S. Immediate effects of core stabilization exercise on β-endorphin and cortisol levels among patients with chronic nonspecific low back pain: A randomized crossover design. *J. Manip. Physiol. Ther.* **2018**, *41*, 181–188. [CrossRef]
51. Williams, K.; Abildso, C.; Steinberg, L.; Doyle, E.; Epstein, B.; Smith, D.; Hobbs, G.; Gross, R.; Kelley, G.; Cooper, L. Evaluation of the effectiveness and efficacy of Iyengar yoga therapy on chronic low back pain. *Spine* **2009**, *34*, 2066–2076. [CrossRef]
52. Stanley, T.D.; Doucouliagos, H.; Ioannidis, J.P.A. Beyond Random Effects: When Small-Study Findings Are More Heterogeneous. *Adv. Methods Pract. Psychol. Sci.* **2022**, *5*, 1–12. [CrossRef]
53. Handley, M.A.; Lyles, C.R.; McCulloch, C.; Cattamanchi, A. Selecting and Improving Quasi-Experimental Designs in Effectiveness and Implementation Research. *Annu. Rev. Public Health* **2018**, *39*, 5–25. [CrossRef] [PubMed]
54. Deeks, J.J.; Dinnes, J.; D'Amico, R.; Sowden, A.J.; Sakarovitch, C.; Song, F.; Petticrew, M.; Altman, D.G. Evaluating non-randomised intervention studies. *Health Technol. Assess* **2003**, *7*, 1–173. [CrossRef] [PubMed]

healthcare

MDPI

Brief Report

The Reliability of the Timed Up and Go Test among Portuguese Elderly

Filipe Rodrigues [1,2], José E. Teixeira [3,4,5] and Pedro Forte [4,5,6,*]

1 ESECS—Polytechnic of Leiria, 2411-901 Leiria, Portugal
2 Life Quality Research Center, 2040-413 Leiria, Portugal
3 Department of Sport Sciences, Polytechnic of Guarda, 6300-559 Guarda, Portugal
4 Department of Sport Sciences, Polytechnic of Bragança, 5300-253 Bragança, Portugal
5 Research Centre in Sports Sciences, Health, and Human Development, 6201-001 Covilhã, Portugal
6 CI-ISCE ISCE Douro, Higher Institute of Educational Sciences of the Douro, 4560-708 Penafiel, Portugal
* Correspondence: pedromiguel.forte@iscedouro.pt

Abstract: Assessment of dynamic balance is typically completed through functional tests, such as the Timed Up and Go (TUG) test, which measures the time it takes for an individual to stand up from a chair, walk a set distance, turn around, and sit back down. This test has been validated in several countries. However, in the Portuguese population there is a gap on testing the reliability of this functional test in a sample of the elderly both living in the community or in nursing homes. Thus, this study aimed at examining the reliability of the TUG in a sample of Portuguese elderly. An Intraclass Correlation Coefficient (ICC) analysis was performed between the first time (T1) and the time score after 16 weeks (T2) in TUG test by 38 males and 79 females aged between 60 and 92 years. The results showed acceptable scores of ICC in community-dwelling and nursing home resident elderly in both moments. In addition, significant differences were found between these groups of older adults, showing that community-dwelling elderly show greater agility and balance capacity compared to those living in nursing homes. Thus, the TUG test can be applied in the Portuguese elderly in both community-dwelling and nursing home resident elderly.

Keywords: older adult; dynamic balance; reliability; measurement

1. Introduction

As the general population continues to age, the preservation of mobility and balance becomes increasingly crucial in sustaining an independent and active lifestyle. Dynamic balance is an important component of physical health in older persons. However, aging is related with a decline in dynamic balance, which can increase the risk of falls and have a detrimental influence on quality of life. Falls can have long-term physical and psychological repercussions, such as disability, fear of falling, and reduced quality of life [1].

The ability of an individual to maintain stability and control while in motion is referred to as dynamic balance [2]. To establish a consistent and efficient movement pattern, sensory input, motor output, and cognitive processes must be coordinated. Dynamic balance is required for daily activities such as walking, ascending stairs, and getting out of a chair, as well as more sophisticated movements such as picking up an object, turning around, and placing it in an elevated area [3]. Multiple physiological systems must collaborate to establish dynamic balance. Through sensory receptors in the skin, muscles, and joints, the somatosensory system gives information about the body's position and movement [4]. The visual system offers input about the environment and helps to adapt motions depending on visual cues. The vestibular system in the inner ear gives information about head movement and direction and plays a critical role in maintaining balance during dynamic movements. Motor output is also critical for achieving dynamic balance. The musculoskeletal system must generate the appropriate force and torque to control movements and maintain postural stability [5]. This requires the coordinated activation of multiple muscle groups, as well as the ability to adjust movements based on feedback from sensory systems. Cognitive processes also play an important role in dynamic balance. Attention, memory, and decision-making are all involved in the planning and execution of movements. The ability to anticipate and respond to environmental cues is essential for successful dynamic balance [6]. Age-related declines in sensory, motor, and cognitive function can all contribute to a loss of dynamic balance, and interventions to improve these functions are essential for maintaining independence and quality of life in older adults [7].

1.1. Assessing Dynamic Balance in the Elderly

Measuring dynamic balance in the older adult population is important for several reasons [8]. First, dynamic balance is an important component of physical function because it helps people to maintain postural stability while walking, turning, and reaching. Impaired dynamic balance can increase the likelihood of falls, which are a leading cause of injury and loss of independence in the elderly. Second, evaluating dynamic balance can assist healthcare providers in tracking changes in physical function over time as well as monitoring the efficacy of programs aimed at improving mobility and balance in older persons. Finally, evaluating dynamic balance in research settings can be a useful tool for identifying risk factors and potential interventions to improve mobility and balance in the aged population [9].

As the population ages, functional assessment techniques are being utilized more frequently to examine the physical performance of older persons. The Timed Up and Go (TUG) test is a functional evaluation instrument described in the literature by Podsiadlo and Richardson in 1991 [10]. The TUG test has received considerable acceptance as a simple, low-cost, and reliable assessment of functional mobility in older persons since its initial publication [8,11]. The test requires an individual to stand up from a chair, walk 2.44 m, turn around, walk back to the chair, and sit down again, with the time taken to complete the test being recorded. The TUG test has been proved to be a valid and reliable assessment of geriatric mobility and fall risk, and it has been widely utilized in clinical and research contexts. It is specifically regarded as a trustworthy and valid instrument for assessing mobility and fall risk in the elderly around the world.

1.2. Balance in Community-Dwelling and Nursing Home Resident Older Adults

There are disparities in dynamic balance between aged people living in the community and those residing in nursing homes, according to extant literature [12]. Nursing home residents frequently have a higher frequency of chronic health issues and functional impairments than community residents. Mobility difficulties, sensory abnormalities, and cognitive decline can all lead to a loss of dynamic balance. Furthermore, nursing home patients may have limited access to exercise and physical activity programs, exacerbating deficits in balance and mobility. Several studies have looked at how dynamic balance differs between community-dwelling older persons and nursing facility residents. One study, for example, discovered that nursing home residents performed much worse on balance than community-dwelling elderly persons [13]. Another study discovered that nursing home patients had considerably lower balance levels than community-dwelling elderly people, indicating poorer dynamic balance [13,14].

1.3. Current Research

Functional test reliability assessments are significant because they provide valuable information on the consistency and reproducibility of test outcomes. The extent to which a test delivers consistent and stable results over time and across testing conditions is referred to as reliability in the context of functional evaluations in the older adult population. Reliability assessments can assist healthcare practitioners and researchers in determining if a test is appropriate for clinical or research purposes, as well as providing insight into the precision and accuracy of test results. Reliable function tests are critical in clinical settings for accurate diagnosis, treatment planning, and monitoring of therapy outcomes. Inconsistent results from an unreliable test might lead to false diagnoses, improper treatment decisions, and a loss of faith in the test results. Reliability analyses are vital in research settings to ensure that study outcomes are accurate and meaningful. If a test is untrustworthy, study results may be difficult to interpret or may not correctly reflect the true impact of an intervention.

There is no scientific evidence to support the reliability of the TUG test in the Portuguese elderly. While it has been used in a number of experimental trials [15,16], comprehensive reliability evaluations are still needed to offer evidence of consistency over time in a sample of Portuguese elderly. Reliability is an important component of validity, which refers to the extent to which a test measures what it is intended to measure. By demonstrating that the TUG test is reliable, the current study can provide evidence that the test is a valid and useful tool for assessing functional mobility in Portuguese older adults living in the community or in nursing homes. Furthermore, there has been no research comparing the findings of the TUG test between elderly people living in the community and those residing in nursing homes. A study comparing the TUG results between elderly individuals living in the community versus those in nursing homes can help to understand differences in functional mobility between these two populations. The purpose of this study was to assess the reliability of the TUG in an elderly population. We also compared the scores of senior people living in the community to those in nursing homes in order to investigate dynamic balance scores and analyze potential discrepancies.

2. Materials and Methods

2.1. Participants

A cross-sectional study with two measurement points was performed as a mean to provide valuable information about the reliability of the TUG over time. By conducting reliability analysis research with two measurement points, researchers can evaluate the consistency and stability of the TUG and determine if the test results are reproducible. The study included a total of 117 participants, comprising 38 males and 79 females, with ages ranging from 60 to 92 years. The mean age of the participants was 77.19 $\pm$ 8.81 years, and the mean body mass index (BMI) was 28.04 $\pm$ 4.11 kg/m^2. The distribution of BMI in the sample was as follows: normal weight (n = 21, 17.9%), overweight (n = 66, 56.4%), and obese (n = 30, 25.7%). Regarding subsamples, the study included a total of 49 community-living older adults (n = 38 females and 11 males), with ages ranging from 58 to 86 years (M = 74.38 $\pm$ 6.33). The study also included a total of 68 nursing home resident older adults (n = 41 females and 27 males), with ages ranging from 56 to 96 years (M = 79.21 $\pm$ 9.78).

Participants in this study were older persons who lived in the community or in nursing homes and met specified inclusion criteria. Participants were eligible if they were 60 or older. If a participant had a known diagnosis of a cognitive disorder or another neurological condition that could impair physical functioning, mobility, or balance, they were excluded. Participants were excluded from participation if they had a history of recent falls, defined as falling twice or more in the previous six months. Participants also had to be able to able to provide informed consent.

2.2. Data Collection Procedures

The data collecting procedures were approved by the Institutional Review Board and adhered to all Helsinki Declaration ethical criteria for human subjects research [17]. To establish a representative sample of the senior population, data for this study were collected in both nursing facilities and community settings. A convenience sampling method was used for data collection, because the researchers could have access to potential participants in both nursing facilities and community settings. Specifically, researchers contacted local nursing homes to obtain approval to conduct the current study. The study was carried out at nursing homes with the help of nursing home employees, who assisted in identifying potential participants based on the inclusion criteria. The researchers then briefed the participants about the goal of the study and received written informed consent. To maintain confidentiality, all data was taken in a private place. In the community, the researchers recruited volunteers through community programs [15,16,18]. Participants who were interested in the study were given information about it and the opportunity to ask questions. They provided written informed permission if they met the inclusion criteria and consented to participate.

Before beginning the TUG exam, participants were told of its purpose and procedures, and they were given the opportunity to ask questions. Participants were told they could opt out of the exam at any point if they felt uncomfortable or unsafe. Two experienced researchers then gave participants a clear and extensive description of the TUG test and demonstrated how to do it. During the exam, participants were allowed to utilize assistive devices they typically use, such as canes or walkers. Participants completed a practice trial to ensure that they understood the instructions and were comfortable doing the test. The researchers thoroughly observed the participants during the test to assure their safety. The experiment was carried out in a clear, open location devoid of obstructions, and the researchers gave physical assistance if needed. Participants were told to complete the exam at a comfortable and safe pace, but feedback was provided before the trial to conduct the test as fast as possible. Participants were given time to rest and recover after the exam, and any concerns or challenges were addressed. The time taken to complete the test was recorded in seconds using a stopwatch (T1). After 16 weeks, the participants completed the same test in the same conditions (T2).

2.3. Statistical Analysis

Prior to conducting the study, a sample size calculation for Intraclass Correlation Coefficient (ICC) analysis was performed using the Arifin calculator [19] to determine the necessary sample size to achieve adequate statistical power. The minimum acceptable reliability was estimated to be 0.70, with a desired significance level of 0.05 and power of 0.95, the calculated minimum sample size was 19. To account for potential dropouts and missing data (10%), to conduct the study, a minimum of 22 participants would need to be recruited. Intraclass Correlation Coefficient (ICC) analysis was conducted to assess the degree of agreement or consistency among multiple measurements of the TUG. The ICC ranges from 0 to 1, with higher values indicating greater agreement or consistency between the measurements. ICC values can be interpreted using commonly-accepted guidelines, such as those proposed by several authors [20,21], where an ICC value of less than 0.40 is considered poor agreement, 0.40–0.59 is fair agreement, 0.60–0.74 is good agreement, and 0.75 or higher is excellent agreement.

Prior to conducting planned *t*-test analyses, sample size calculation was performed using the Soper calculator [22] to determine the necessary sample size to achieve adequate statistical power. The anticipated effect size was estimated to be 0.5 based on previous research in the field [20,21]. With a desired alpha level of 0.05 and power of 0.95, the calculated minimum sample size was 64. To account for potential dropouts and missing data, to conduct the study, a minimum of 75 participants would need to be recruited.

3. Results

The results of the ICC analysis are reported in Table 1. As it stands, the ICC for both groups displayed acceptable scores. We also calculated bivariate correlations for additional evidence. The results showed that the correlation between T1 and T2 for community-dwelling elderly was $r = 0.97$, and the same correlation for nursing home resident older adults was $r = 0.82$. Thus, the results support the reliability of the TUG among elderly from two different resident homes. Considering the results from the *t*-test analyses, as theoretically expected, community-dwelling elderly displayed significant better scores than nursing home resident older adults in the T1 ($F = 51.46$; $t\ [1, 115] = -6.68$; $p < 0.05$) and T2 ($F = 36.04$; $t\ [1, 115] = -5.45$; $p < 0.05$) moments.

Table 1. Means, standard deviations and inter-class correlation coefficients.

Community-Dwelling Elderly (n = 49)			Nursing Home Resident Elderly (n = 68)		
T1	T2	ICC	T1	T2	ICC
4.65 (0.81)	4.48 (0.84)	0.97	18.90 (14.89)	16.11 (14.89)	0.82

Notes: Data in T1 and T2 are reported in Mean and Standard Deviation; brackets = standard deviation; ICC = Intra-Class Correlation coefficients.

4. Discussion

The purpose of the present study was to assess the reliability of the TUG in a Portuguese elderly population. We also compared the scores of senior people living in the community to those in nursing homes in order to investigate dynamic balance scores and analyze potential differences. The results showed that the TUG displayed acceptable scores of ICC both in community-dwelling and nursing home resident elderly. In addition, significant differences were found between these groups of older adults, showing that community-dwelling elderly show greater agility and balance capacity compared to those living in nursing homes.

In the current study, the reliability of the TUG test was similar or close to those reported in previously published studies [23–25]. Many studies have used the ICC to assess the reliability of the TUG test. Shumway-Cook et al. (2000), for example, reported an ICC value of 0.98 for the TUG test in a sample of American elderly. Similar ICC results are reported in Japanese elderly [26] and Swedish older adults [25]. This implies that the test is very reliable and that results acquired on several occasions are likely to be consistent. In fact, the results displayed in the validation study of the TUG test by Podsiadlo and Richardson [10] that revealed an ICC value of 0.98 for the TUG test, confirming the high reliability of this test.

Statistically significant differences were found between community-dwelling elderly and those living in nursing homes regarding the TUG test results. These results are in accordance with previous literature [9,13]. According to studies, community-dwelling older persons have faster TUG test results than nursing facility residents. Verghese et al. [27] discovered that community-dwelling older persons had a mean TUG test result of 9.20 s, while nursing facility residents had a mean TUG test result of 19.20 s, which are similar in the present study. TUG test results from community-dwelling elderly and nursing home resident elderly were compared in an Italian study, and nursing home resident elderly had considerably longer TUG test times than community-dwelling elderly [28]. Another Brazilian study revealed that nursing home residents had greater TUG test times than community-dwelling seniors [29].

This disparity in TUG test results between community-dwelling elderly and those living in nursing homes could be attributed to a variety of factors, including disparities in overall health, mobility, and functional independence. The elderly in residential care homes are often frail. They have several diagnoses, a high medicine intake, a lack of general strength, and are prone to illness and disease. This participation of multiple systems probably generates sources of unpredictability and can be linked to a condition of unstable impairment or frailty [28]. Frailty is a disease or syndrome resulting from a multisystem decline in reserve capacity to the extent that a number of physiological systems are close to, or have passed, the threshold of symptomatic clinical failure. Frailty is thought to be the underlying cause of unbalance [29]. It should be noted that the TUG test is only one measure of functional mobility; other tests may be more effective for assessing functional mobility in other populations. While interpreting TUG test findings, it is also crucial to consider individual variances in health state, mobility, and functional independence.

Limitations and Agenda for Future Research

The current findings should be restricted to healthy Portuguese elderly living in the community or nursing homes who can walk at least 10 m with or without a walking aid. Additionally, the degree of plantar flexor tone was not quantified, which may have influenced the current findings. We also did not measure agility and balance using other validated measures (e.g., Berg Balance Scale; Fall Efficacy Scale) that could serve for concurrent validity analysis. Information about premedical chronic disease history and magnitude may influence results. Gender influence was not explored in this study because there were fewer male elderly.

5. Conclusions

The results of the present study showed that the TUG presented acceptable scores of ICC both in community-dwelling and nursing home resident elderly. In addition, significant differences were found between these groups of older adults, showing that community-dwelling elderly show greater agility and balance capacity compared to those living in nursing homes. It is a quick and easy test that assesses how long it takes an individual to get out of a chair, walk 2.44 m, turn around, walk back to the chair, and sit down. The TUG test is a low-cost instrument for assessing functional ability in the elderly. It requires minimal equipment and can be carried out by a variety of healthcare professionals (e.g., exercise physiologists, nurses), reducing the requirement for specialist equipment or personnel.

Author Contributions: Conceptualization, F.R.; methodology, J.E.T.; validation, P.F.; formal analysis, J.E.T.; investigation, P.F.; resources, J.E.T.; writing—original draft preparation, F.R.; writing—review and editing, J.E.T.; supervision, P.F.; project administration, F.R.; funding acquisition, F.R. and P.F. All authors have read and agreed to the published version of the manuscript.

Funding: This research was funded by national funds through the Portuguese Foundation for Science and Technology, I.P., grant number UID/04748/2020 and grant number UID04045/2020.

Institutional Review Board Statement: The study was conducted according to the guidelines of the Declaration of Helsinki and approved by the Scientific Board of the IP Leiria (nº = CE/IPLEIRIA/59/2022 approved on 14 December 2022).

Informed Consent Statement: Informed consent was obtained from all subjects involved in the study. Written informed consent has been obtained from the patients to publish this paper.

Data Availability Statement: Data are available upon request from the contact author.

Acknowledgments: We thank all older adults for their participation in this study.

Conflicts of Interest: The authors declare no conflict of interest.

References

1. Schoene, D.; Heller, C.; Aung, Y.N.; Sieber, C.C.; Kemmler, W.; Freiberger, E. A Systematic Review on the Influence of Fear of Falling on Quality of Life in Older People: Is There a Role for Falls? *Clin. Interv. Aging* **2019**, *14*, 701–719. [CrossRef] [PubMed]
2. Dunsky, A.; Zeev, A.; Netz, Y. Balance Performance Is Task Specific in Older Adults. *BioMed Res. Int.* **2017**, *2017*, 6987017. [CrossRef]
3. Shumway-Cook, A.; Silver, I.F.; LeMier, M.; York, S.; Cummings, P.; Koepsell, T.D. Effectiveness of a Community-Based Multifactorial Intervention on Falls and Fall Risk Factors in Community-Living Older Adults: A Randomized, Controlled Trial. *J. Gerontol. A Biol. Sci. Med. Sci.* **2007**, *62*, 1420–1427. [CrossRef] [PubMed]
4. Prochazka, A. Sensory Control of Normal Movement and of Movement Aided by Neural Prostheses. *J. Anat.* **2015**, *227*, 167–177. [CrossRef] [PubMed]
5. Rodrigues, F.; Domingos, C.; Monteiro, D.; Morouço, P. A Review on Aging, Sarcopenia, Falls, and Resistance Training in Community-Dwelling Older Adults. *Int. J. Environ. Res. Public Health* **2022**, *19*, 874. [CrossRef] [PubMed]
6. Fu, Z.; Sajad, A.; Errington, S.P.; Schall, J.D.; Rutishauser, U. Neurophysiological Mechanisms of Error Monitoring in Human and Non-Human Primates. *Nat. Rev. Neurosci.* **2023**, *24*, 153–172. [CrossRef] [PubMed]
7. Campos, J.L.; Marusic, U.; Mahoney, J.R. Editorial: The Intersection of Cognitive, Motor, and Sensory Processing in Aging: Links to Functional Outcomes, Volume I. *Front. Aging Neurosci.* **2022**, *14*, 963. [CrossRef]
8. Rikli, R.E.; Jones, C.J. Development and Validation of Criterion-Referenced Clinically Relevant Fitness Standards for Maintaining Physical Independence in Later Years. *Gerontologist* **2013**, *53*, 255–267. [CrossRef]
9. Piotrowski, A.; Cole, J. Clinical Measures of Balance and Functional Assessment in Elderly Persons. *Aust. J. Physiother.* **1994**, *40*, 183–188. [CrossRef]

10. Podsiadlo, D.; Richardson, S. The Timed "Up & Go": A Test of Basic Functional Mobility for Frail Elderly Persons. *J. Am. Geriatr. Soc.* **1991**, *39*, 142–148. [CrossRef]
11. Barry, E.; Galvin, R.; Keogh, C.; Horgan, F.; Fahey, T. Is the Timed Up and Go Test a Useful Predictor of Risk of Falls in Community Dwelling Older Adults: A Systematic Review and Meta-Analysis. *BMC Geriatr.* **2014**, *14*, 14. [CrossRef]
12. Kang, K.-H.; White, K.N.; Hayes, W.C.; Snow, C.M. Agility and Balance Differ Between Older Community and Retirement Facility Residents. *J. Appl. Gerontol.* **2004**, *23*, 457–468. [CrossRef]
13. Bischoff, H.A.; Stähelin, H.B.; Monsch, A.U.; Iversen, M.D.; Weyh, A.; Von Dechend, M.; Akos, R.; Conzelmann, M.; Dick, W.; Theiler, R. Identifying a Cut-off Point for Normal Mobility: A Comparison of the Timed "up and Go" Test in Community-Dwelling and Institutionalised Elderly Women. *Age Ageing* **2003**, *32*, 315–320. [CrossRef]
14. Monteiro, A.M.; Rodrigues, S.; Matos, S.; Teixeira, J.E.; Barbosa, T.M.; Forte, P. The Effects of 32 Weeks of Multicomponent Training with Different Exercises Order in Elderly Women's Functional Fitness and Body Composition. *Medicina* **2022**, *58*, 628. [CrossRef]
15. Rodrigues, F.; Monteiro, A.M.; Forte, P.; Morouço, P. Effects of Muscle Strength, Agility, and Fear of Falling on Risk of Falling in Older Adults. *Int. J. Environ. Res. Public Health* **2023**, *20*, 4945. [CrossRef]
16. Rodrigues, F.; Amaro, N.; Matos, R.; Mendes, D.; Monteiro, D.; Morouço, P. The Impact of an Exercise Intervention Using Low-Cost Equipment on Functional Fitness in the Community-Dwelling Older Adults: A Pilot Study. *Front. Physiol.* **2022**, *13*, 2211. [CrossRef]
17. World Medical Association. World Medical Association Declaration of Helsinki: Ethical Principles for Medical Research Involving Human Subjects. *JAMA* **2013**, *310*, 2191–2194. [CrossRef]
18. Rodrigues, F.; Jacinto, M.; Figueiredo, N.; Monteiro, A.M.; Forte, P. Effects of a 24-Week Low-Cost Multicomponent Exercise Program on Health-Related Functional Fitness in the Community-Dwelling Aged and Older Adults. *Medicina* **2023**, *59*, 371. [CrossRef]
19. Arifin, W.N. Sample Size Calculator. 2022. Available online: https://wnarifin.github.io/ssc_web.html (accessed on 10 February 2023).
20. Koo, T.K.; Li, M.Y. A Guideline of Selecting and Reporting Intraclass Correlation Coefficients for Reliability Research. *J. Chiropr. Med.* **2016**, *15*, 155–163. [CrossRef]
21. Landis, J.R.; Koch, G.G. The Measurement of Observer Agreement for Categorical Data. *Biometrics* **1977**, *33*, 159–174. [CrossRef]
22. Soper, D.S. A-Priori Sample Size Calculator for Structural Equation Models. 2020. Available online: https://www.danielsoper.com/statcalc/calculator.aspx?id=89 (accessed on 30 January 2023).
23. Christopher, A.; Kraft, E.; Olenick, H.; Kiesling, R.; Doty, A. The Reliability and Validity of the Timed Up and Go as a Clinical Tool in Individuals with and without Disabilities across a Lifespan: A Systematic Review. *Disabil. Rehabil.* **2021**, *43*, 1799–1813. [CrossRef] [PubMed]
24. Shumway-Cook, A.; Brauer, S.; Woollacott, M. Predicting the Probability for Falls in Community-Dwelling Older Adults Using the Timed Up & Go Test. *Phys. Ther.* **2000**, *80*, 896–903. [PubMed]
25. Nordin, E.; Rosendahl, E.; Lundin-Olsson, L. Timed "Up & Go" Test: Reliability in Older People Dependent in Activities of Daily Living—Focus on Cognitive State. *Phys. Ther.* **2006**, *86*, 646–655. [CrossRef] [PubMed]
26. Asai, T.; Oshima, K.; Fukumoto, Y.; Yonezawa, Y.; Matsuo, A.; Misu, S. Association of Fall History with the Timed Up and Go Test Score and the Dual Task Cost: A Cross-Sectional Study among Independent Community-Dwelling Older Adults. *Geriatr. Gerontol. Int.* **2018**, *18*, 1189–1193. [CrossRef]
27. Verghese, J.; Lipton, R.B.; Hall, C.B.; Kuslansky, G.; Katz, M.J.; Buschke, H. Abnormality of Gait as a Predictor of Non-Alzheimer's Dementia. *N. Engl. J. Med.* **2002**, *347*, 1761–1768. [CrossRef]
28. Mulas, I.; Putzu, V.; Asoni, G.; Viale, D.; Mameli, I.; Pau, M. Clinical Assessment of Gait and Functional Mobility in Italian Healthy and Cognitively Impaired Older Persons Using Wearable Inertial Sensors. *Aging Clin. Exp. Res.* **2021**, *33*, 1853–1864. [CrossRef]
29. Oliveira-Zmuda, G.G.; Soldera, C.L.C.; Jovanov, E.; Bós, Â.J.G. Timed Up and Go Test Phases as Predictors of Future Falls in Community-Dwelling Older Adults. *Fisioter. Mov.* **2022**, *35*, e35142. [CrossRef]

MDPI AG
Grosspeteranlage 5
4052 Basel
Switzerland
Tel.: +41 61 683 77 34

Healthcare Editorial Office
E-mail: healthcare@mdpi.com
www.mdpi.com/journal/healthcare

www.ingramcontent.com/pod-product-compliance
Lightning Source LLC
Chambersburg PA
CBHW062101220926
51850CB00010B/2849
* 9 7 8 3 7 2 5 8 7 8 3 5 2 *